12 Month Workout Plan

Complete

Improve Fitness,

Build Muscles,

Increase Strength

Andrea Raimondi

CONTENTS

Introduction 4
Break-in phase (8 weeks) 6
Strength phase (8 weeks) 16
Recovery phase (4 weeks) 25
Hypertrophy phase (12 weeks) 30
Strength Phase #2 44
Hypertrophy Phase #2 53
Aerobic Activity 66
How to continue 68
Lockdown 69
Motivation 75
BONUS Lunch-time Workout 77

For a complete course on bodybuilding and body recomposition check out my book on Amazon

https://www.amazon.com/dp/B08RK235ZX

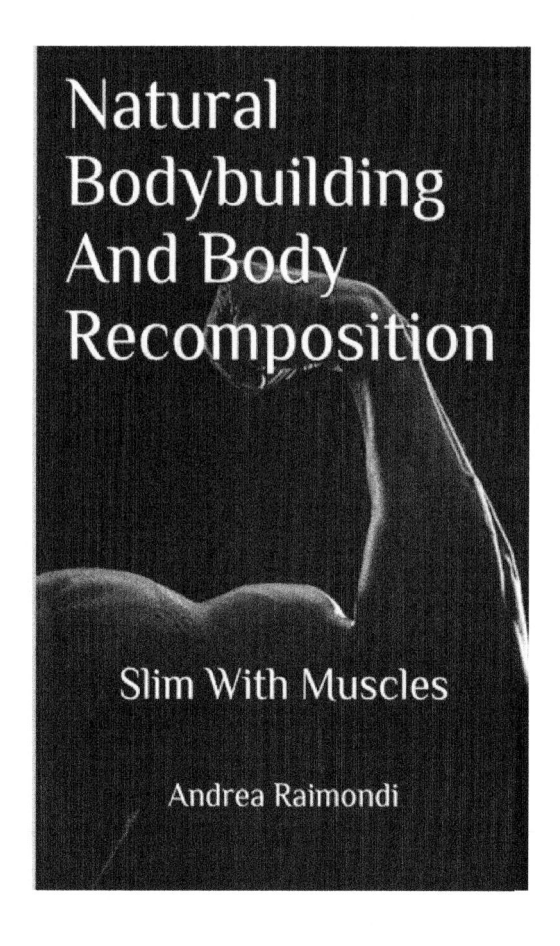

Introduction

Below you will find the detail of my training protocol lasting a total of 52 weeks, 12 months of training, at the end of which it is possible to continue, resuming a certain phase that better fit your needs. This macrocycle is divided into four main phases: a break-in or **adaptation phase** lasting 8 weeks suitable for those who have just started training or for those who resume activity after a period of rest. This is followed by an 8 weeks **strength phase** in which we try to increase overall strength. After the strength phase, very expensive for the body, follows a **recovery phase** lasting 4 weeks. The last mesocycle of the protocol consists of the **hypertrophy phase** lasting 12 weeks, in which the workouts will be aimed at gaining muscle mass. At the end of the period of hypertrophy it is good to insert a recovery period of another 4 weeks. At this point you have to decide based on your goals and restart with a cycle of strength or with another cycle of hypertrophy. In first case restart 8 weeks of **strength** phase, 4 weeks of recovery and another 8 weeks of **strength** phase. If your goal is hypertrophy you can continue with 12 weeks of hypertrophy protocol and 4 weeks of recovery protocol.

Keep track of your exercises using my webapp, designed for Personal Trainer.

Follow the trend of your workout or body parameters with graphs.

PT-Manager.com

https://www.pt-manager.com/start/index_eng.html

FREE TRIAL AVAILABLE!

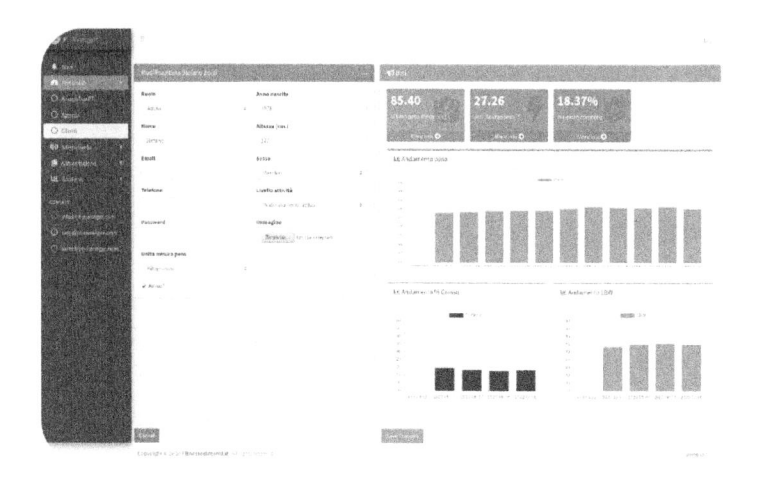

Break-in phase (8 weeks)

This phase is designed for those who have never trained with weights or for those who have not trained for a long time.

Those who have been training for at least 6 months can use this phase as a preparation for the next ones or start directly with the strength phase.

The protocol provides for an 8 week mesocycle divided into two sections.

There are three days of training in each week.

The first section has the main purpose of learning the movements for the various exercises. All major muscle groups are trained in each session.

They are "Full body" workouts in which the weight do not have to be heavy and the repetitions are quite high, from 15 to 20 per set, with rests of about 1 minute between sets.

It is important to start very gradually to allow the body to adapt to the effort without incurring injuries or annoying pains that can block your desire to train.

Always do one or two sets of warm-ups with a low load before each exercise.

Every week increase the maximum weight used in the training setss.

Phase two, also with full body sessions and lasting four weeks, includes weeks with light loads and others with heavier loads.

Throughout the initial phase, but more generally during training, you must try to maintain a "clean" movement, focusing on the muscle you are working on.

Keep an execution speed (TUT) of 2 seconds during the concentric phase and 2 seconds in the eccentric phase. About the weight to be lifted: it varies according to your initial state of form and experience as well as your initial strength. To make the use of the cards universal, I adopted the system relating to the maximum repetition, or rather the maximum number of repetitions that you can perform with a given weight. For example, if 3 sets @ 8-10RM is indicated, it means that you must use a weight that allows you to perform a maximum of 10 repetitions correctly and not less than 8, if then in another card for the same exercise that number is lowers, i.e. find @ 5-7RM means that with the weight used you can perform a maximum of 7 repetitions, i.e. the load is heavier than the first indication.

Initial phase. Section 1. Week 1
Perceived effort level 6

DAY	MUSCLES	EXERCISES
Monday	Full Body	Dumbbell bench press [3 sets @ 15-20RM] Dumbbell military press [3 sets @ 15-20RM] Dumbbell bent over row [3 sets @ 15-20RM] Dumbbell curl [3 sets @ 15-20RM] Cable pushdown [3 sets @ 15-20RM] Leg curl [3 sets @ 15-20RM] Squat [3 sets @ 15-20RM] Crunch [3 sets @ 15-20RM] Calf raise [3 sets @ 15-20RM]
Tuesday	Rest	
Wednesday	Full Body	Dumbbell bench press [3 sets @ 15-20RM] Dumbbell military press [3 sets @ 15-20RM] Dumbbell bent over row [3 sets @15-20RM] Dumbbell curl [3 sets @ 15-20RM] Cable pushdown [3 sets @ 15-20RM] Leg curl [3 sets @ 15-20RM] Squat [3 sets @ 15-20RM] Crunch [3 sets @ 15-20RM] Calf raise [3 sets @ 15-20RM]
Thursday	Rest	
Friday	Full Body	Dumbbell bench press [3 sets @ 15-20RM] Dumbbell military press [3 sets @ 15-20RM] Dumbbell bent over row [3 sets @ 15-20RM] Dumbbell curl [3 sets @ 15-20RM] Cable pushdown [3 sets @ 15-20RM] Leg curl [3 sets @ 15-20RM] Squat [3 sets @ 15-20RM] Crunch [3 sets @ 15-20RM] Calf raise [3 sets @ 15-20RM]
Saturday	Rest	Aerobic Activity
Sunday	Rest	

Initial phase. Section 1. Week 2
Perceived effort level 7, add weight each set

DAY	MUSCLES	EXERCISES
Monday	Full Body	Dumbbell bench press [3 sets @ 15-20RM] Dumbbell military press [3 sets @ 15-20RM] Dumbbell bent over row [3 sets @ 15-20RM] Dumbbell curl [3 sets @ 15-20RM] Cable pushdown [3 sets @ 15-20RM] Leg curl [3 sets @ 15-20RM] Squat [3 sets @ 15-20RM] Crunch [3 sets @ 15-20RM] Calf raise [3 sets @ 15-20RM]
Tuesday	Rest	
Wednesday	Full Body	Dumbbell bench press [3 sets @ 15-20RM] Dumbbell military press [3 sets @ 15-20RM] Dumbbell bent over row [3 sets @ 15-20RM] Dumbbell curl [3 sets @ 15-20RM] Cable pushdown [3 sets @ 15-20RM] Leg curl [3 sets @ 15-20RM] Squat [3 sets @ 15-20RM] Crunch [3 sets @ 15-20RM] Calf raise [3 sets @ 15-20RM]
Thursday	Rest	
Friday	Full Body	Dumbbell bench press [3 sets @ 15-20RM] Dumbbell military press [3 sets @ 15-20RM] Dumbbell bent over row [3 sets @ 15-20RM] Dumbbell curl [3 sets @ 15-20RM] Cable pushdown [3 sets @ 15-20RM] Leg curl [3 sets @ 15-20RM] Squat [3 sets @ 15-20RM] Crunch [3 sets @ 15-20RM] Calf raise [3 sets @ 15-20RM]
Saturday	Rest	Aerobic Activity
Sunday	Rest	

Initial phase. Section 1. Week 3
Perceived effort level 8, add weight each set

DAY	MUSCLES	EXERCISES
Monday	Full Body	Dumbbell bench press [3 sets @ 15-20RM] Dumbbell military press [3 sets @ 15-20RM] Dumbbell bent over row [3 sets @ 15-20RM] Dumbbell curl [3 sets @ 15-20RM] Cable pushdown [3 sets @ 15-20RM] Leg curl [3 sets @ 15-20RM] Squat [3 sets @ 15-20RM] Crunch [3 sets @ 15-20RM] Calf raise [3 sets @ 15-20RM]
Tuesday	Rest	
Wednesday	Full Body	Dumbbell bench press [3 sets @ 15-20RM] Dumbbell military press [3 sets @ 15-20RM] Dumbbell bent over row [3 sets @ 15-20RM] Dumbbell curl [3 sets @ 15-20RM] Cable pushdown [3 sets @ 15-20RM] Leg curl [3 sets @ 15-20RM] Squat [3 sets @ 15-20RM] Crunch [3 sets @ 15-20RM] Calf raise [3 sets @ 15-20RM]
Thursday	Rest	
Friday	Full Body	Dumbbell bench press [3 sets @ 15-20RM] Dumbbell military press [3 sets @ 15-20RM] Dumbbell bent over row [3 sets @ 15-20RM] Dumbbell curl [3 sets @ 15-20RM] Cable pushdown [3 sets @ 15-20RM] Leg curl [3 sets @ 15-20RM] Squat [3 sets @ 15-20RM] Crunch [3 sets @ 15-20RM] Calf raise [3 sets @ 15-20RM]
Saturday	Rest	Aerobic Activity
Sunday	Rest	

Initial phase. Section 1. Week 4
Perceived effort level 6

DAY	MUSCLES	EXERCISES
Monday	Full Body	Dumbbell bench press [3 sets @ 15-20RM] Dumbbell military press [3 sets @ 15-20RM] Dumbbell bent over row [3 sets @ 15-20RM] Dumbbell curl [3 sets @ 15-20RM] Cable pushdown [3 sets @ 15-20RM] Leg curl [3 sets @ 15-20RM] Squat [3 sets @ 15-20RM] Crunch [3 sets @ 15-20RM] Calf raise [3 sets @ 15-20RM]
Tuesday	Rest	
Wednesday	Full Body	Dumbbell bench press [3 sets @ 15-20RM] Dumbbell military press [3 sets @ 15-20RM] Dumbbell bent over row [3 sets @ 15-20RM] Dumbbell curl [3 sets @ 15-20RM] Cable pushdown [3 sets @ 15-20RM] Leg curl [3 sets @ 15-20RM] Squat [3 sets @ 15-20RM] Crunch [3 sets @ 15-20RM] Calf raise [3 sets @ 15-20RM]
Thursday	Rest	
Friday	Full Body	Dumbbell bench press [3 sets @ 15-20RM] Dumbbell military press [3 sets @ 15-20RM] Dumbbell bent over row [3 sets @ 15-20RM] Dumbbell curl [3 sets @ 15-20RM] Cable pushdown [3 sets @ 15-20RM] Leg curl [3 sets @ 15-20RM] Squat [3 sets @ 15-20RM] Crunch [3 sets @ 15-20RM] Calf raise [3 sets @ 15-20RM]
Saturday	Rest	Aerobic Activity
Sunday	Rest	

Initial phase. Section 2. Week 5
Perceived effort level 6

DAY	MUSCLES	EXERCISES
Monday	Full Body	Dumbbell bench press [3 sets @ 15-20RM] Dumbbell military press [3 sets @ 15-20RM] Low pulley row [3 sets @ 15-20RM] Dumbbell curl [3 sets @ 15-20RM] Cable pushdown [3 sets @ 15-20RM] Leg curl [3 sets @ 15-20RM] Leg extension [3 sets @ 15-20RM] Crunch [3 sets @ 15-20RM] Calf raise [3 sets @ 15-20RM]
Tuesday	Rest	
Wednesday	Full Body	Dumbbell bench press [3 sets @ 15-20RM] Dumbbell military press [3 sets @ 15-20RM] Low pulley row [3 sets @ 15-20RM] Dumbbell curl [3 sets @ 15-20RM] Cable pushdown [3 sets @ 15-20RM] Leg curl [3 sets @ 15-20RM] Leg extension [3 sets @ 15-20RM] Crunch [3 sets @ 15-20RM] Calf raise [3 sets @ 15-20RM]
Thursday	Rest	
Friday	Full Body	Dumbbell bench press [3 sets @ 15-20RM] Dumbbell military press [3 sets @ 15-20RM] Low pulley row [3 sets @ 15-20RM] Dumbbell curl [3 sets @ 15-20RM] Cable pushdown [3 sets @ 15-20RM] Leg curl [3 sets @ 15-20RM] Leg extension [3 sets @ 15-20RM] Crunch [3 sets @ 15-20RM] Calf raise [3 sets @ 15-20RM]
Saturday	Rest	Aerobic Activity
Sunday	Rest	

Initial phase. Section 2. Week 6
Perceived effort level 7

DAY	MUSCLES	EXERCISES
Monday	Full Body	Dumbbell bench press [3 sets @ 10-12RM] Dumbbell military press [3 sets @ 10-12RM] Low pulley row [3 sets @ 10-12RM] Dumbbell curl [3 sets @ 10-12RM] Cable pushdown [3 sets @ 10-12RM] Leg curl [3 sets @ 10-12RM] Leg extension [3 sets @ 10-12RM] Crunch [3 sets @ 10-12RM] Calf raise [3 sets @ 10-12RM]
Tuesday	Rest	
Wednesday	Full Body	Dumbbell bench press [3 sets @ 10-12RM] Dumbbell military press [3 sets @ 10-12RM] Low pulley row [3 sets @ 10-12RM] Dumbbell curl [3 sets @ 10-12RM] Cable pushdown [3 sets @ 10-12RM] Leg curl [3 sets @ 10-12RM] Leg extension [3 sets @ 10-12RM] Crunch [3 sets @ 10-12RM] Calf raise [3 sets @ 10-12RM]
Thursday	Rest	
Friday	Full Body	Dumbbell bench press [3 sets @ 10-12RM] Dumbbell military press [3 sets @ 10-12RM] Low pulley row [3 sets @ 10-12RM] Dumbbell curl [3 sets @ 10-12RM] Cable pushdown [3 sets @ 10-12RM] Leg curl [3 sets @ 10-12RM] Leg extension [3 sets @ 10-12RM] Crunch [3 sets @ 10-12RM] Calf raise [3 sets @ 10-12RM]
Saturday	Rest	Aerobic Activity
Sunday	Rest	

Initial phase. Section 2. Week 7
Perceived effort level 7

DAY	MUSCLES	EXERCISES
Monday	Full Body	Dumbbell bench press [3 sets @ 8-10RM] Dumbbell military press [3 sets @ 8-10RM] Low pulley row [3 sets @ 8-10RM] Dumbbell curl [3 sets @ 8-10RM] Cable pushdown [3 sets @ 8-10RM] Leg curl [3 sets @ 8-10RM] Leg extension [3 sets @ 8-10RM] Crunch [3 sets @ 8-10RM] Calf raise [3 sets @ 8-10RM]
Tuesday	Rest	
Wednesday	Full Body	Dumbbell bench press [3 sets @ 8-10RM] Dumbbell military press [3 sets @ 8-10RM] Low pulley row [3 sets @ 8-10RM] Dumbbell curl [3 sets @ 8-10RM] Cable pushdown [3 sets @ 8-10RM] Leg curl [3 sets @ 8-10RM] Leg extension [3 sets @ 8-10RM] Crunch [3 sets @ 8-10RM] Calf raise [3 sets @ 8-10RM]
Thursday	Rest	
Friday	Full Body	Dumbbell bench press [3 sets @ 8-10RM] Dumbbell military press [3 sets @ 8-10RM] Low pulley row [3 sets @ 8-10RM] Dumbbell curl [3 sets @ 8-10RM] Cable pushdown [3 sets @ 8-10RM] Leg curl [3 sets @ 8-10RM] Leg extension [3 sets @ 8-10RM] Crunch [3 sets @ 8-10RM] Calf raise [3 sets @ 8-10RM]
Saturday	Rest	Aerobic Activity
Sunday	Rest	

Initial phase. Section 2. Week 8
Perceived effort level 7

DAY	MUSCLES	EXERCISES
Monday	Full Body	Dumbbell bench press [3 sets @ 15-20RM] Dumbbell military press [3 sets @ 15-20RM] Low pulley row [3 sets @ 15-20RM] Dumbbell curl [3 sets @ 15-20RM] Cable pushdown [3 sets @ 15-20RM] Leg curl [3 sets @ 15-20RM] Leg extension [3 sets @ 15-20RM] Crunch [3 sets @ 15-20RM] Calf raise [3 sets @ 15-20RM]
Tuesday	Rest	
Wednesday	Full Body	Dumbbell bench press [3 sets @ 15-20RM] Dumbbell military press [3 sets @ 15-20RM] Low pulley row [3 sets @ 15-20RM] Dumbbell curl [3 sets @ 15-20RM] Cable pushdown [3 sets @ 15-20RM] Leg curl [3 sets @ 15-20RM] Leg extension [3 sets @ 15-20RM] Crunch [3 sets @ 15-20RM] Calf raise [3 sets @ 15-20RM]
Thursday	Rest	
Friday	Full Body	Dumbbell bench press [3 sets @ 15-20RM] Dumbbell military press [3 sets @ 15-20RM] Low pulley row [3 sets @ 15-20RM] Dumbbell curl [3 sets @ 15-20RM] Cable pushdown [3 sets @ 15-20RM] Leg curl [3 sets @ 15-20RM] Leg extension [3 sets @ 15-20RM] Crunch [3 sets @ 15-20RM] Calf raise [3 sets @ 15-20RM]
Saturday	Rest	Aerobic Activity
Sunday	Rest	

Strength phase (8 weeks)

This phase is divided into two mesocycles of four weeks each, in which you train with high loads and low repetitions, the rests between one sets and the next are lengthened up to 2-3 minutes.
In the first mesocycle you train three days a week in full body, in the second at least four days but with split routines. Remember to keep the correct movement, the weight always in control.

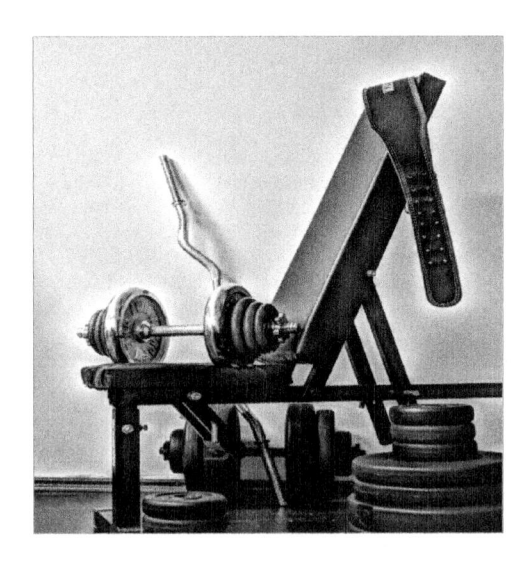

Strength phase. Section 1. Week 1
Perceived effort level 8, add weight each set.

DAY	MUSCLES	EXERCISES
Monday	Full Body	Bench press [3 sets @ 5-6 RM] Military press [3 sets @ 15-6 RM] Low pulley row [3 sets @ 5-6 RM] Dumbbell curl [3 sets @ 5-6 RM] Cable pushdown [3 sets @ 5-6 RM] Leg curl [3 sets @ 5-6 RM] Squat [3 sets @ 5-6 RM] Crunch [3 sets @ 15-20RM]
Tuesday	Rest	
Wednesday	Full Body	Bench press [3 sets @ 5-6 RM] Military press [3 sets @ 15-6 RM] Low pulley row [3 sets @ 5-6 RM] Dumbbell curl [3 sets @ 5-6 RM] Cable pushdown [3 sets @ 5-6 RM] Leg curl [3 sets @ 5-6 RM] Squat [3 sets @ 5-6 RM] Crunch [3 sets @ 15-20RM]
Thursday	Rest	
Friday	Full Body	Bench press [3 sets @ 5-6 RM] Military press [3 sets @ 15-6 RM] Low pulley row [3 sets @ 5-6 RM] Dumbbell curl [3 sets @ 5-6 RM] Cable pushdown [3 sets @ 5-6 RM] Leg curl [3 sets @ 5-6 RM] Squat [3 sets @ 5-6 RM] Crunch [3 sets @ 15-20RM]
Saturday	Rest	Aerobic Activity
Sunday	Rest	

Strength phase. Section 1. Week 2
Perceived effort level 8, add weight each set.

DAY	MUSCLES	EXERCISES
Monday	Full Body	Bench press [3 sets @ 3-5 RM] Military press [3 sets @ 3-5 RM] Low pulley row [3 sets @ 3-5 RM] Dumbbell curl [3 sets @ 3-5 RM] Cable pushdown [3 sets @ 3-5 RM] Leg curl [3 sets @ 3-5 RM] Squat [3 sets @ 3-5 RM] Crunch [3 sets @ 15-20RM]
Tuesday	Rest	
Wednesday	Full Body	Bench press [3 sets @ 3-5 RM] Military press [3 sets @ 3-5 RM] Low pulley row [3 sets @ 3-5 RM] Dumbbell curl [3 sets @ 3-5 RM] Cable pushdown [3 sets @ 3-5 RM] Leg curl [3 sets @ 3-5 RM] Squat [3 sets @ 3-5 RM] Crunch [3 sets @ 15-20RM]
Thursday	Rest	
Friday	Full Body	Bench press [3 sets @ 3-5 RM] Military press [3 sets @ 3-5 RM] Low pulley row [3 sets @ 3-5 RM] Dumbbell curl [3 sets @ 3-5 RM] Cable pushdown [3 sets @ 3-5 RM] Leg curl [3 sets @ 3-5 RM] Squat [3 sets @ 3-5 RM] Crunch [3 sets @ 15-20RM]
Saturday	Rest	Aerobic Activity
Sunday	Rest	

Strength phase. Section 1. Week 3
Perceived effort level 8, add weight each set.

DAY	MUSCLES	EXERCISES
Monday	Full Body	Bench press [3 sets @ 1-3 RM] Military press [3 sets @ 1-3 RM] Low pulley row [3 sets @ 1-3 RM] Dumbbell curl [3 sets @ 1-3 RM] Cable pushdown [3 sets @ 1-3 RM] Leg curl [3 sets @ 1-3 RM] Squat [3 sets @ 1-3 RM] Crunch [3 sets @ 15-20RM]
Tuesday	Rest	
Wednesday	Full Body	Bench press [3 sets @ 1-3 RM] Military press [3 sets @ 1-3 RM] Low pulley row [3 sets @ 1-3 RM] Dumbbell curl [3 sets @ 1-3 RM] Cable pushdown [3 sets @ 1-3 RM] Leg curl [3 sets @ 1-3 RM] Squat [3 sets @ 1-3 RM] Crunch [3 sets @ 15-20RM]
Thursday	Rest	
Friday	Full Body	Bench press [3 sets @ 1-3 RM] Military press [3 sets @ 1-3 RM] Low pulley row [3 sets @ 1-3 RM] Dumbbell curl [3 sets @ 1-3 RM] Cable pushdown [3 sets @ 1-3 RM] Leg curl [3 sets @ 1-3 RM] Squat [3 sets @ 1-3 RM] Crunch [3 sets @ 15-20RM]
Saturday	Rest	Aerobic Activity
Sunday	Rest	

Strength phase. Section 1. Week 4
Perceived effort level 7.

DAY	MUSCLES	EXERCISES
Monday	Full Body	Bench press [3 sets @ 10-12 RM] Military press [3 sets @ 10-12 RM] Low pulley row [3 sets @ 10-12 RM] Dumbbell curl [3 sets @ 10-12 RM] Cable pushdown [3 sets @ 10-12 RM] Leg curl [3 sets @ 10-12 RM] Squat [3 sets @ 10-12 RM] Crunch [3 sets @ 15-20RM]
Tuesday	Rest	
Wednesday	Full Body	Bench press [3 sets @ 10-12 RM] Military press [3 sets @ 10-12 RM] Low pulley row [3 sets @ 10-12 RM] Dumbbell curl [3 sets @ 10-12 RM] Cable pushdown [3 sets @ 10-12 RM] Leg curl [3 sets @ 10-12 RM] Squat [3 sets @ 10-12 RM] Crunch [3 sets @ 15-20RM]
Thursday	Rest	
Friday	Full Body	Bench press [3 sets @ 10-12 RM] Military press [3 sets @ 10-12 RM] Low pulley row [3 sets @ 10-12 RM] Dumbbell curl [3 sets @ 10-12 RM] Cable pushdown [3 sets @ 10-12 RM] Leg curl [3 sets @ 10-12 RM] Squat [3 sets @ 10-12 RM] Crunch [3 sets @ 15-20RM]
Saturday	Rest	Aerobic Activity
Sunday	Rest	

Strength phase. Section 2. Week 5
Perceived effort level 8, add weight each set.

DAY	MUSCLES	EXERCISES
Monday	Upper Body	Bench press [3 sets @ 6-8 RM] Military press [3 sets @ 6-8 RM] Dumbbell flyes [3 sets @ 6-8 RM] Lat machine [3 sets @ 6-8 RM] Dumbbell curl [3 sets @ 6-8 RM] Cable pushdown [3 sets @ 6-8 RM]
Tuesday	Lower Body	Leg curl [3 sets @ 6-8 RM] Squat [3 sets @ 6-8 RM] Calf raise [3 sets @ 6-8 RM] Crunch [3 sets @ 15-20RM]
Wednesday	Rest	
Thursday	Upper Body	Bench press [3 sets @ 6-8 RM] Military press [3 sets @ 6-8 RM] Lateral raises [3 sets @ 6-8 RM] Lat machine [3 sets @ 6-8 RM] Dumbbell curl [3 sets @ 6-8 RM] Cable pushdown [3 sets @ 6-8 RM]
Friday	Lower Body	Leg curl [3 sets @ 6-8 RM] Squat [3 sets @ 6-8 RM] Calf raise [3 sets @ 6-8 RM] Crunch [3 sets @ 15-20RM]
Saturday	Rest	Aerobic Activity
Sunday	Rest	

Strength phase. Section 2. Week 6
Perceived effort level 8, add weight each set.

DAY	MUSCLES	EXERCISES
Monday	Upper Body	Bench press [3 sets @ 3-5 RM] Military press [3 sets @ 3-5 RM] Dumbbell flyes [3 sets @ 3-5 RM] Lat machine [3 sets @ 3-5 RM] Dumbbell curl [3 sets @ 3-5 RM] Cable pushdown [3 sets @ 3-5 RM]
Tuesday	Lower Body	Leg curl [3 sets @ 3-5 RM] Squat [3 sets @ 3-5 RM] Calf raise [3 sets @ 3-5 RM] Crunch [3 sets @ 15-20RM]
Wednesday	Rest	
Thursday	Upper Body	Bench press [3 sets @ 3-5 RM] Military press [3 sets @ 3-5 RM] Lateral raises [3 sets @3-5 RM] Lat machine [3 sets @ 3-5 RM] Dumbbell curl [3 sets @ 3-5 RM] Cable pushdown [3 sets @ 3-5 RM]
Friday	Lower Body	Leg curl [3 sets @ 3-5 RM] Squat [3 sets @ 3-5 RM] Calf raise [3 sets @ 3-5 RM] Crunch [3 sets @ 15-20RM]
Saturday	Rest	Aerobic Activity
Sunday	Rest	

Strength phase. Section 2. Week 7
Perceived effort level 9, add weight each set.

DAY	MUSCLES	EXERCISES
Monday	Upper Body	Bench press [3 sets @ 2-3 RM] Military press [3 sets @ 2-3 RM] Dumbbell flyes [3 sets @ 2-3 RM] Lat machine [3 sets @ 2-3 RM] Dumbbell curl [3 sets @ 2-3 RM] Cable pushdown [3 sets @ 2-3 RM]
Tuesday	Lower Body	Leg curl [3 sets @ 2-3 RM] Squat [3 sets @ 2-3 RM] Calf raise [3 sets @ 2-3 RM] Crunch [3 sets @ 15-20RM]
Wednesday	Rest	
Thursday	Upper Body	Bench press [3 sets @ 2-3 RM] Military press [3 sets @ 2-3 RM] Lateral raises [3 sets @2-3 RM] Lat machine [3 sets @ 2-3 RM] Dumbbell curl [3 sets @ 2-3 RM] Cable pushdown [3 sets @ 2-3 RM]
Friday	Lower Body	Leg curl [3 sets @ 2-3 RM] Squat [3 sets @ 2-3 RM] Calf raise [3 sets @ 2-3 RM] Crunch [3 sets @ 15-20RM]
Saturday	Rest	Aerobic Activity
Sunday	Rest	

Strength phase. Section 2. Week 8
Perceived effort level 7, add weight each set.

DAY	MUSCLES	EXERCISES
Monday	Upper Body	Bench press [3 sets @ 10-12 RM] Military press [3 sets @ 10-12 RM] Dumbbell flyes [3 sets @ 10-12RM] Lat machine [3 sets @ 10-12 RM] Dumbbell curl [3 sets @ 10-12 RM] Cable pushdown [3 sets @ 10-12 RM]
Tuesday	Lower Body	Leg curl [3 sets @ 10-12 RM] Squat [3 sets @ 10-12 RM] Calf raise [3 sets @ 10-12 RM] Crunch [3 sets @ 15-20RM]
Wednesday	Rest	
Thursday	Upper Body	Bench press [3 sets @ 10-12 RM] Military press [3 sets @ 10-12 RM] Dumbbell flyes [3 sets @ 10-12 RM] Lat machine [3 sets @ 10-12 RM] Dumbbell curl [3 sets @ 10-12 RM] Cable pushdown [3 sets @ 10-12 RM]
Friday	Lower Body	Leg curl [3 sets @ 10-12 RM] Squat [3 sets @ 10-12 RM] Calf raise [3 sets @ 10-12 RM] Crunch [3 sets @ 15-20RM]
Saturday	Rest	Aerobic Activity
Sunday	Rest	

Recovery phase (4 weeks)

In this mesocycle we increase the repetitions by decreasing the maximum weight used, this gives the body the time it needs to recover after the strength phase, which was a period of intense work. At the same time, we reduce the recovery time between one set and the next to increase metabolic work. This procedure can also be used in protocols for definition or slimming in combination with a low-calorie diet.

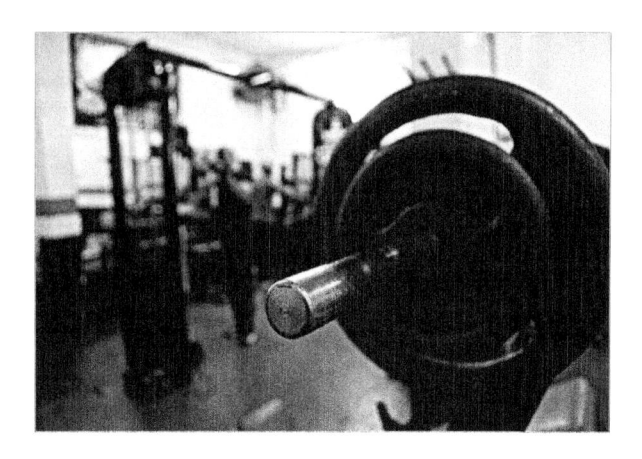

Recovery phase. Week 1
Perceived efford 7, rest 30-45'' between sets

DAY	MUSCLES	EXERCISES
Monday	Full Body	Dumbbell bench press [3 sets @ 15-20RM] Dumbbell military press [3 sets @ 15-20RM] Low pulley row [3 sets @ 15-20RM] Dumbbell curl [3 sets @ 15-20RM] Cable pushdown [3 sets @ 15-20RM] Leg curl [3 sets @ 15-20RM] Leg extension [3 sets @ 15-20RM] Crunch [3 sets @ 15-20RM] Calf raise [3 sets @ 15-20RM]
Tuesday	Rest	
Wednesday	Full Body	Dumbbell flyes [3 sets @ 10-12RM] Lateral raises [3 sets @ 110-12RM] Low pulley row [3 sets @ 10-12RM] Dumbbell curl [3 sets @ 10-12RM] Cable pushdown [3 sets @ 10-12RM] Leg curl [3 sets @ 10-12RM] Leg extension [3 sets @ 10-12RM] Crunch [3 sets @ 10-12RM] Calf raise [3 sets @ 10-12RM]
Thursday	Rest	Aerobic Activity
Friday	Full Body	Dumbbell bench press [3 sets @ 15-20RM] Dumbbell military press [3 sets @ 15-20RM] Low pulley row [3 sets @ 15-20RM] Dumbbell curl [3 sets @ 15-20RM] Cable pushdown [3 sets @ 15-20RM] Leg curl [3 sets @ 15-20RM] Leg extension [3 sets @ 15-20RM] Crunch [3 sets @ 15-20RM] Calf raise [3 sets @ 15-20RM]
Saturday	Rest	Aerobic Activity
Sunday	Rest	

Recovery phase. Week 2
Perceived efford 6-7, rest 30-45'' between sets

DAY	MUSCLES	EXERCISES
Monday	Full Body	Dumbbell bench press [3 sets @ 15-20RM] Dumbbell military press [3 sets @ 15-20RM] Lat machine [3 sets @ 15-20RM] Dumbbell curl [3 sets @ 15-20RM] Cable pushdown [3 sets @ 15-20RM] Leg curl [3 sets @ 15-20RM] Leg press [3 sets @ 15-20RM] Crunch [3 sets @ 15-20RM] Calf raise [3 sets @ 15-20RM]
Tuesday	Rest	
Wednesday	Full Body	Dumbbell flyes [3 sets @ 10-12RM] Lateral raises [3 sets @ 110-12RM] Low pulley row [3 sets @ 10-12RM] Dumbbell curl [3 sets @ 10-12RM] Cable pushdown [3 sets @ 10-12RM] Leg curl [3 sets @ 10-12RM] Leg extension [3 sets @ 10-12RM] Crunch [3 sets @ 10-12RM] Calf raise [3 sets @ 10-12RM]
Thursday	Rest	Aerobic Activity
Friday	Full Body	Dumbbell bench press [3 sets @ 15-20RM] Dumbbell military press [3 sets @ 15-20RM] Lat machine [3 sets @ 15-20RM] Dumbbell curl [3 sets @ 15-20RM] Cable pushdown [3 sets @ 15-20RM] Leg curl [3 sets @ 15-20RM] Leg press [3 sets @ 15-20RM] Crunch [3 sets @ 15-20RM] Calf raise [3 sets @ 15-20RM]
Saturday	Rest	Aerobic Activity
Sunday	Rest	

Recovery phase. Week 3
Perceived efford 6-7, rest 30-45'' between sets

DAY	MUSCLES	EXERCISES
Monday	Full Body	Dumbbell bench press [3 sets @ 15-20RM] Dumbbell military press [3 sets @ 15-20RM] Low pulley row [3 sets @ 15-20RM] Dumbbell curl [3 sets @ 15-20RM] Cable pushdown [3 sets @ 15-20RM] Leg curl [3 sets @ 15-20RM] Leg extension [3 sets @ 15-20RM] Crunch [3 sets @ 15-20RM] Calf raise [3 sets @ 15-20RM]
Tuesday	Rest	
Wednesday	Full Body	Dumbbell flyes [3 sets @ 10-12RM] Lateral raises [3 sets @ 110-12RM] Low pulley row [3 sets @ 10-12RM] Dumbbell curl [3 sets @ 10-12RM] Cable pushdown [3 sets @ 10-12RM] Leg curl [3 sets @ 10-12RM] Leg extension [3 sets @ 10-12RM] Crunch [3 sets @ 10-12RM] Calf raise [3 sets @ 10-12RM]
Thursday	Rest	Aerobic Activity
Friday	Full Body	Dumbbell bench press [3 sets @ 15-20RM] Dumbbell military press [3 sets @ 15-20RM] Low pulley row [3 sets @ 15-20RM] Dumbbell curl [3 sets @ 15-20RM] Cable pushdown [3 sets @ 15-20RM] Leg curl [3 sets @ 15-20RM] Leg extension [3 sets @ 15-20RM] Crunch [3 sets @ 15-20RM] Calf raise [3 sets @ 15-20RM]
Saturday	Rest	Aerobic Activity
Sunday	Rest	

Recovery phase. Week 4
Perceived efford 7, rest 30-45'' between sets

DAY	MUSCLES	EXERCISES
Monday	Full Body	Dumbbell bench press [3 sets @ 15-20RM] Dumbbell military press [3 sets @ 15-20RM] Lat machine [3 sets @ 15-20RM] Dumbbell curl [3 sets @ 15-20RM] Cable pushdown [3 sets @ 15-20RM] Leg curl [3 sets @ 15-20RM] Leg press [3 sets @ 15-20RM] Crunch [3 sets @ 15-20RM] Calf raise [3 sets @ 15-20RM]
Tuesday	Rest	
Wednesday	Full Body	Dumbbell flyes [3 sets @ 15-20RM] Lateral raises [3 sets @ 15-20RM] Low pulley row [3 sets @ 15-20RM] Dumbbell curl [3 sets @ 15-20RM] Cable pushdown [3 sets @ 15-20RM] Leg curl [3 sets @ 15-20RM] Leg extension [3 sets @ 15-20RM] Crunch [3 sets @ 15-20RM] Calf raise [3 sets @ 15-20RM]
Thursday	Rest	Aerobic Activity
Friday	Full Body	Dumbbell bench press [3 sets @ 15-20RM] Dumbbell military press [3 sets @ 15-20RM] Lat machine [3 sets @ 15-20RM] Dumbbell curl [3 sets @ 15-20RM] Cable pushdown [3 sets @ 15-20RM] Leg curl [3 sets @ 15-20RM] Leg press [3 sets @ 15-20RM] Crunch [3 sets @ 15-20RM] Calf raise [3 sets @ 15-20RM]
Saturday	Rest	Aerobic Activity
Sunday	Rest	

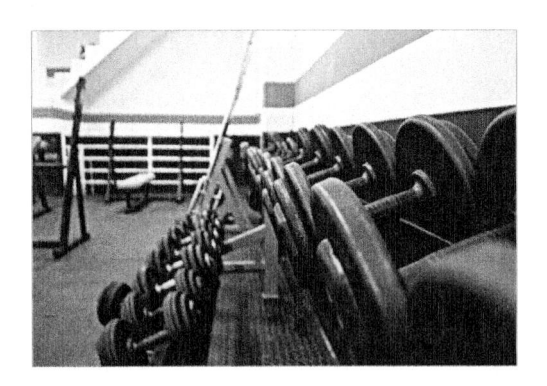

Hypertrophy phase (12 weeks)

In this phase we will seek maximum muscle development. It is divided into three mesocycles of four weeks.

Medium to high loads will be used to allow 6 to 12 repetitions; rest between sets will be 60-90 seconds.

The repetitions must always be performed in full control of the movement.

The first mesocycle is in full body over three days. The second and third mesocycles are based on a 5-day split routine.

The weight will be increased after each week excluding the last week of each mesocycle to allow adequate recovery without losing muscle tone.

Hypertrophy phase. Mesocycle 1. Week 1.

DAY	MUSCLES	EXERCISES
Monday	Full Body	Dumbbell bench press [3 sets @ 10-12RM] Dumbbell military press [3 sets @ 10-12RM] Low pulley row [3 sets @ 10-12RM] Dumbbell curl [3 sets @ 10-12RM] Cable pushdown [3 sets @ 10-12RM] Leg curl [3 sets @ 10-12RM] Leg extension [3 sets @ 10-12RM] Crunch [3 sets @ 10-12RM] Calf raise [3 sets @ 10-12RM]
Tuesday	Rest	
Wednesday	Full Body	Dumbbell flyes [3 sets @ 10-12RM] Lateral raises [3 sets @ 10-12RM] Lat machine [3 sets @ 10-12RM] Dumbbell curl [3 sets @ 10-12RM] Cable pushdown [3 sets @ 10-12RM] Leg curl [3 sets @ 10-12RM] Leg extension [3 sets @ 10-12RM] Crunch [3 sets @ 10-12RM] Calf raise [3 sets @ 10-12RM]
Thursday	Rest	
Friday	Full Body	Dumbbell bench press [3 sets @ 10-12RM] Dumbbell military press [3 sets @ 10-12RM] Low pulley row [3 sets @ 10-12RM] Dumbbell curl [3 sets @ 10-12RM] Cable pushdown [3 sets @ 10-12RM] Leg curl [3 sets @ 10-12RM] Leg extension [3 sets @ 10-12RM] Crunch [3 sets @ 10-12RM] Calf raise [3 sets @ 10-12RM]
Saturday	Rest	Aerobic Activity
Sunday	Rest	

Hypertrophy phase. Mesocycle 1. Week 2.

DAY	MUSCLES	EXERCISES
Monday	Full Body	Dumbbell bench press [3 sets @ 8-10RM] Dumbbell military press [3 sets @ 1 8-10RM] Low pulley row [3 sets @ 8-10RM] Dumbbell curl [3 sets @ 8-10RM] Cable pushdown [3 sets @ 8-10RM] Leg curl [3 sets @ 8-10RM] Leg extension [3 sets @ 8-10RM] Crunch [3 sets @ 8-10RM] Calf raise [3 sets @ 8-10RM]
Tuesday	Rest	
Wednesday	Full Body	Dumbbell flyes [3 sets @ 8-10RM] Lateral raises [3 sets @ 8-10RM] Lat machine [3 sets @ 8-10RM] Dumbbell curl [3 sets @ 8-10RM] Cable pushdown [3 sets @ 8-10RM] Leg curl [3 sets @ 8-10RM] Leg extension [3 sets @ 8-10RM] Crunch [3 sets @ 8-10RM] Calf raise [3 sets @ 8-10RM]
Thursday	Rest	
Friday	Full Body	Dumbbell bench press [3 sets @ 8-10RM] Dumbbell military press [3 sets @ 1 8-10RM] Low pulley row [3 sets @ 8-10RM] Dumbbell curl [3 sets @ 8-10RM] Cable pushdown [3 sets @ 8-10RM] Leg curl [3 sets @ 8-10RM] Leg extension [3 sets @ 8-10RM] Crunch [3 sets @ 8-10RM] Calf raise [3 sets @ 8-10RM]
Saturday	Rest	
Sunday	Rest	

Hypertrophy phase. Mesocycle 1. Week 3.

Loads are increased and repetitions reduced, always with maximum control of movement. Recovery of 60 sec. between one set and another.

DAY	MUSCLES	EXERCISES
Monday	Full Body	Dumbbell bench press [3 sets @ 6-8RM] Dumbbell military press [3 sets @ 6-8RM] Low pulley row [3 sets @ 6-8RM] Dumbbell curl [3 sets @ 6-8 RM] Cable pushdown [3 sets @ 6-8RM] Leg curl [3 sets @ 6-8RM] Leg extension [3 sets @ 6-8RM] Crunch [3 sets @ 6-8RM] Calf raise [3 sets @ 6-8RM]
Tuesday	Rest	
Wednesday	Full Body	Dumbbell flyes [3 sets @ 6-8RM] Lateral raises [3 sets @ 6-8RM] Lat machine [3 sets @ 6-8RM] Dumbbell curl [3 sets @ 6-8RM] Cable pushdown [3 sets @ 6-8RM] Leg curl [3 sets @ 6-8RM] Leg extension [3 sets @ 6-8RM] Crunch [3 sets @ 6-8RM] Calf raise [3 sets @ 6-8RM]
Thursday	Rest	
Friday	Full Body	Dumbbell bench press [3 sets @ 6-8RM] Dumbbell military press [3 sets @ 6-8RM] Low pulley row [3 sets @ 6-8RM] Dumbbell curl [3 sets @ 6-8 RM] Cable pushdown [3 sets @ 6-8RM] Leg curl [3 sets @ 6-8RM] Leg extension [3 sets @ 6-8RM] Crunch [3 sets @ 6-8RM] Calf raise [3 sets @ 6-8RM]
Saturday	Rest	Aerobic Activity
Sunday	Rest	

Hypertrophy phase. Mesocycle 1. Week 4.
Lower the weights, increase repetitions, rest 45-60''

DAY	MUSCLES	EXERCISES
Monday	Full Body	Dumbbell bench press [3 sets @ 10-12RM] Dumbbell military press [3 sets @ 10-12RM] Low pulley row [3 sets @ 10-12RM] Dumbbell curl [3 sets @ 10-12RM] Cable pushdown [3 sets @ 10-12RM] Leg curl [3 sets @ 10-12RM] Leg extension [3 sets @ 10-12RM] Crunch [3 sets @ 10-12RM] Calf raise [3 sets @ 10-12RM]
Tuesday	Rest	
Wednesday	Full Body	Dumbbell flyes [3 sets @ 10-12RM] Lateral raises [3 sets @ 10-12RM] Lat machine [3 sets @ 10-12RM] Dumbbell curl [3 sets @ 10-12RM] Cable pushdown [3 sets @ 10-12RM] Leg curl [3 sets @ 10-12RM] Leg extension [3 sets @ 10-12RM] Crunch [3 sets @ 10-12RM] Calf raise [3 sets @ 10-12RM]
Thursday	Rest	
Friday	Full Body	Dumbbell bench press [3 sets @ 10-12RM] Dumbbell military press [3 sets @ 10-12RM] Low pulley row [3 sets @ 10-12RM] Dumbbell curl [3 sets @ 10-12RM] Cable pushdown [3 sets @ 10-12RM] Leg curl [3 sets @ 10-12RM] Leg extension [3 sets @ 10-12RM] Crunch [3 sets @ 10-12RM] Calf raise [3 sets @ 10-12RM]
Saturday	Rest	Aerobic Activity
Sunday	Rest	

Hypertrophy phase. Mesocycle 2. Week 5.

DAY	MUSCLES	EXERCISES
Monday	Chest, Back, Legs, Abs	Dumbbell bench press [4 sets @ 10-12RM] Dumbbell flyes [4 sets @ 10-12RM] Low pulley row [4 sets @ 10-12RM] Leg curl [4 sets @ 10-12RM] Crunch [4 sets @ 10-12RM]
Tuesday	Shoulders, Legs, Abs	Military press [4 sets @ 10-12RM] Lateral raises [4 sets @ 10-12RM] Rear lateral raises [4 sets @ 10-12RM] Leg extension [4 sets @ 10-12RM] Leg Press [4 sets @ 10-12RM] Calf raise [4 sets @ 10-12RM] Crunch [4 sets @ 10-12RM]
Wednesday	Arms, Abs	Dumbbell curl [3 sets @ 10-12RM] Cable pushdown [3 sets @ 10-12RM] Crunch [4 sets @ 10-12RM]
Thursday	Chest, Back, Legs, Abs	Dumbbell bench press [4 sets @ 10-12RM] Dumbbell flyes [4 sets @ 10-12RM] Lat machine [4 sets @ 10-12RM] Leg curl [4 sets @ 10-12RM] Crunch [4 sets @ 10-12RM]
Friday	Shoulders, Legs, Abs	Military press [4 sets @ 10-12RM] Lateral raises [4 sets @ 10-12RM] Rear lateral raises [4 sets @ 10-12RM] Leg extension [4 sets @ 10-12RM] Leg Press [4 sets @ 10-12RM] Calf raise [4 sets @ 10-12RM] Crunch [4 sets @ 10-12RM]
Saturday	Rest	Aerobic Activity
Sunday	Rest	

Hypertrophy phase. Mesocycle 2. Week 6. Increase weights, rest 60-90''

DAY	MUSCLES	EXERCISES
Monday	Chest, Back, Legs, Abs	Dumbbell bench press [4 sets @ 8-10RM] Dumbbell flyes [4 sets @ 8-10RM] Low pulley row [4 sets @ 8-10RM] Leg curl [4 sets @ 8-10RM] Crunch [4 sets @ 15-20RM]
Tuesday	Shoulders, Legs, Abs	Military press [4 sets @ 8-10RM] Lateral raises [4 sets @ 8-10RM] Rear lateral raises [4 sets @ 8-10RM] Leg extension [4 sets @ 8-10RM] Leg Press [4 sets @ 8-10RM] Calf raise [4 sets @ 8-10RM] Crunch [4 sets @ 15-20RM]
Wednesday	Arms, Abs	Dumbbell curl [4 sets @ 8-10RM] Cable pushdown [4 sets @ 8-10RM] Crunch [4 sets @ 8-10RM]
Thursday	Chest, Back, Legs, Abs	Dumbbell bench press [4 sets @ 8-10RM] Dumbbell flyes [4 sets @ 8-10RM] Lat machine [4 sets @ 8-10RM] Leg curl [4 sets @ 8-10RM] Crunch [4 sets @ 15-20RM]
Friday	Shoulders, Legs, Abs	Military press [4 sets @ 8-10RM] Lateral raises [4 sets @ 8-10RM] Rear lateral raises [4 sets @ 8-10RM] Leg extension [4 sets @ 8-10RM] Leg Press [4 sets @ 8-10RM] Calf raise [4 sets @ 8-10RM] Crunch [4 sets @ 15-20RM]
Saturday	Rest	Aerobic Activity
Sunday	Rest	

Hypertrophy phase. Mesocycle 2. Week 7.
Increase sets using high weights, rest 60-90''

DAY	MUSCLES	EXERCISES
Monday	Chest, Back, Legs, Abs	Dumbbell bench press [5 sets @ 8-10 RM] Dumbbell flyes [5 sets @ 8-10 RM] Low pulley row [5 sets @ 8-10 RM] Leg curl [5 sets @ 8-10 RM] Crunch [4 sets @ 15-20 RM]
Tuesday	Shoulders, Legs, Abs	Military press [5 sets @ 8-10 RM] Lateral raises [5 sets @ 8-10 RM] Rear lateral raises [5 sets @ 8-10 RM] Leg extension [5 sets @ 8-10 RM] Leg Press [4 sets @ 8-10RM] Calf raise [5 sets @ 8-10 RM] Crunch [4 sets @ 15-20RM]
Wednesday	Arms, Abs	Dumbbell curl [5 sets @ 8-10RM] Cable pushdown [5 sets @ 8-10RM] Crunch [4 sets @ 15-20RM]
Thursday	Chest, Back, Legs, Abs	Dumbbell bench press [5 sets @ 8-10 RM] Dumbbell flyes [5 sets @ 8-10 RM] Lat machine [5 sets @ 8-10 RM] Leg curl [5 sets @ 8-10 RM] Crunch [4 sets @ 15-20 RM]
Friday	Shoulders, Legs, Abs	Military press [5 sets @ 8-10 RM] Lateral raises [5 sets @ 8-10 RM] Rear lateral raises [5 sets @ 8-10 RM] Leg extension [5 sets @ 8-10 RM] Leg Press [4 sets @ 8-10RM] Calf raise [5 sets @ 8-10 RM] Crunch [4 sets @ 15-20RM]
Saturday	Rest	Aerobic Activity
Sunday	Rest	

Hypertrophy phase. Mesocycle 2. Week 8.
Lower weights, increase repetitions, rest 45-60''

DAY	MUSCLES	EXERCISES
Monday	Chest, Back, Legs, Abs	Dumbbell bench press [4 sets @ 15-20RM] Dumbbell flyes [4 sets @ 15-20RM] Low pulley row [4 sets @ 15-20RM] Leg curl [4 sets @ 15-20RM] Crunch [4 sets @ 15-20RM]
Tuesday	Shoulders, Legs, Abs	Military press [4 sets @ 15-20RM] Lateral raises [4 sets @ 15-20RM] Rear lateral raises [4 sets @ 15-20RM] Leg extension [4 sets @ 15-20RM] Leg Press [4 sets @ 15-20RM] Calf raise [4 sets @ 15-20RM] Crunch [4 sets @ 15-20RM]
Wednesday	Arms, Abs	Dumbbell curl [3 sets @ 15-20RM] Cable pushdown [3 sets @ 15-20RM] Crunch [4 sets @ 15-20RM]
Thursday	Chest, Back, Legs, Abs	Dumbbell bench press [4 sets @ 15-20RM] Dumbbell flyes [4 sets @ 15-20RM] Lat machine [4 sets @ 15-20RM] Leg curl [4 sets @ 15-20RM] Crunch [4 sets @ 15-20RM]
Friday	Shoulders, Legs, Abs	Military press [4 sets @ 15-20RM] Lateral raises [4 sets @ 15-20RM] Rear lateral raises [4 sets @ 15-20RM] Leg extension [4 sets @ 15-20RM] Leg Press [4 sets @ 15-20RM] Calf raise [4 sets @ 15-20RM] Crunch [4 sets @ 15-20RM]
Saturday	Rest	Aerobic Activity
Sunday	Rest	

Hypertrophy phase. Mesocycle 3. Week 9.
Superset and triset. Rest di 60-90''

DAY	MUSCLES	EXERCISES
Monday	Chest, Back, Legs, Abs	Dumbbell bench press [4 sets @ 8-10 RM] superset with Dumbbell flyes [4 sets @ 8-10 RM] Low pulley row [4 sets @ 8-10 RM] Leg curl [4 sets @ 8-10 RM] Crunch [4 sets @ 15-20 RM]
Tuesday	Shoulders, Legs, Abs	Military press [4 sets @ 8-10 RM] triset with Lateral raises [4 sets @ 8-10 RM] e Rear lateral raises [4 sets @ 8-10 RM] Leg extension [4 sets @ 8-10 RM] superset with Leg Press [4 sets @ 8-10RM] Calf raise [4 sets @ 8-10 RM] Crunch [4 sets @ 15-20RM]
Wednesday	Arms, Abs	Dumbbell curl [4 sets @ 8-10RM] Cable pushdown [4 sets @ 8-10RM] Crunch [4 sets @ 15-20RM]
Thursday	Chest, Back, Legs, Abs	Dumbbell bench press [4 sets @ 8-10 RM] superset with Dumbbell flyes [4 sets @ 8-10 RM] Lat machine [4 sets @ 8-10 RM] Leg curl [4 sets @ 8-10 RM] Crunch [4 sets @ 15-20 RM]
Friday	Shoulders, Legs, Abs	Military press [4 sets @ 8-10 RM] triset with Lateral raises [4 sets @ 8-10 RM] e Rear lateral raises [4 sets @ 8-10 RM] Leg extension [4 sets @ 8-10 RM] superset with Leg Press [4 sets @ 8-10RM] Calf raise [4 sets @ 8-10 RM] Crunch [4 sets @ 15-20RM]
Saturday	Rest	Aerobic Activity
Sunday	Rest	

Hypertrophy phase. Mesocycle 3. Week 10.

DAY	MUSCLES	EXERCISES
Monday	Chest, Back, Legs, Abs	Dumbbell bench press [5 sets @ 8-10 RM] superset with Dumbbell flyes [5 sets @ 8-10 RM] Low pulley row [5 sets @ 8-10 RM] Leg curl [5 sets @ 8-10 RM] Crunch [4 sets @ 15-20 RM]
Tuesday	Shoulders, Legs, Abs	Military press [5 sets @ 8-10 RM] triset with Lateral raises [5 sets @ 8-10 RM] e Rear lateral raises [5 sets @ 8-10 RM] Leg extension [5 sets @ 8-10 RM] superset Leg Press [4 sets @ 8-10RM] Calf raise [5 sets @ 8-10 RM] Crunch [4 sets @ 15-20RM]
Wednesday	Arms, Abs	Dumbbell curl [5 sets @ 8-10RM] Cable pushdown [5 sets @ 8-10RM] Crunch [4 sets @ 15-20RM]
Thursday	Chest, Back, Legs, Abs	Dumbbell bench press [5 sets @ 8-10 RM] superset with Dumbbell flyes [5 sets @ 8-10 RM] Lat machine[5 sets @ 8-10 RM] Leg curl [5 sets @ 8-10 RM] Crunch [4 sets @ 15-20 RM]
Friday	Shoulders, Legs, Abs	Military press [5 sets @ 8-10 RM] triset with Lateral raises [5 sets @ 8-10 RM] e Rear lateral raises [5 sets @ 8-10 RM] Leg extension [5 sets @ 8-10 RM] superset with Leg Press [4 sets @ 8-10RM] Calf raise [5 sets @ 8-10 RM] Crunch [4 sets @ 15-20RM]
Saturday	Rest	Aerobic Activity
Sunday	Rest	

Hypertrophy phase. Mesocycle 3. Week 11. Increase weight. Rest 90-120''

DAY	MUSCLES	EXERCISES
Monday	Chest, Back, Legs, Abs	Dumbbell bench press [4 sets @ 6-8 RM] superset with Dumbbell flyes [4 sets @ 6-8 RM] Low pulley row [4 sets @ 6-8 RM] Leg curl [4 sets @ 6-8 RM] Crunch [4 sets @ 15-20 RM]
Tuesday	Shoulders, Legs, Abs	Military press [4 sets @ 6-8 RM] triset with Lateral raises [4 sets @ 6-8 RM] e Rear lateral raises [4 sets @ 6-8 RM] Leg extension [4 sets @ 6-8 RM] superset with Leg Press [4 sets @ 6-8 RM] Calf raise [4 sets @ 6-8 RM] Crunch [4 sets @ 15-20RM]
Wednesday	Arms, Abs	Dumbbell curl [4 sets @ 6-8 RM] Cable pushdown [4 sets @ 6-8 RM] Crunch [4 sets @ 15-20RM]
Thursday	Chest, Back, Legs, Abs	Dumbbell bench press [4 sets @ 6-8 RM] superset with Dumbbell flyes [4 sets @ 6-8 RM] Lat machine [4 sets @ 6-8 RM] Leg curl [4 sets @ 6-8 RM] Crunch [4 sets @ 15-20 RM]
Friday	Shoulders, Legs, Abs	Military press [4 sets @ 6-8 RM] triset with Lateral raises [4 sets @ 6-8 RM] e Rear lateral raises [4 sets @ 6-8 RM] Leg extension [4 sets @ 6-8 RM] superset with Leg Press [4 sets @ 6-8 RM] Calf raise [4 sets @ 6-8 RM] Crunch [4 sets @ 15-20RM]
Saturday	Rest	Aerobic Activity
Sunday	Rest	

Hypertrophy phase. Mesocycle 3. Week 12.
Lower weight. Rest 60-90''

DAY	MUSCLES	EXERCISES
Monday	Chest, Back, Legs, Abs	Dumbbell bench press [4 sets @ 15-20RM] Dumbbell flyes [4 sets @ 15-20RM] Low pulley row [4 sets @ 15-20RM] Leg curl [4 sets @ 15-20RM] Crunch [4 sets @ 15-20RM]
Tuesday	Shoulders, Legs, Abs	Military press [4 sets @ 15-20RM] Lateral raises [4 sets @ 15-20RM] Rear lateral raises [4 sets @ 15-20RM] Leg extension [4 sets @ 15-20RM] Leg Press [4 sets @ 15-20RM] Calf raise [4 sets @ 15-20RM] Crunch [4 sets @ 15-20RM]
Wednesday	Arms, Abs	Dumbbell curl [3 sets @ 15-20RM] Cable pushdown [3 sets @ 15-20RM] Crunch [4 sets @ 15-20RM]
Thursday	Chest, Back, Legs, Abs	Dumbbell bench press [4 sets @ 15-20RM] Dumbbell flyes [4 sets @ 15-20RM] Lat machine [4 sets @ 15-20RM] Leg curl [4 sets @ 15-20RM] Crunch [4 sets @ 15-20RM]
Friday	Shoulders, Legs, Abs	Military press [4 sets @ 15-20RM] Lateral raises [4 sets @ 15-20RM] Rear lateral raises [4 sets @ 15-20RM] Leg extension [4 sets @ 15-20RM] Leg Press [4 sets @ 15-20RM] Calf raise [4 sets @ 15-20RM] Crunch [4 sets @ 15-20RM]
Saturday	Rest	Aerobic Activity
Sunday	Rest	

After the 12 weeks of the hypertrophy protocol and having checked our physical form with respect to the desired goals, we can continue with the metabolic adaptation protocol for a four-week mesocycle. These four weeks can lead to an increase in muscle definition when conducted with a calorie deficit. Or we can decide to stop training for 2-3 weeks and then restart with a phase of strength or hypertrophy. This stop period could coincide with the summer holidays in which you reach the maximum of muscle development and your condition.

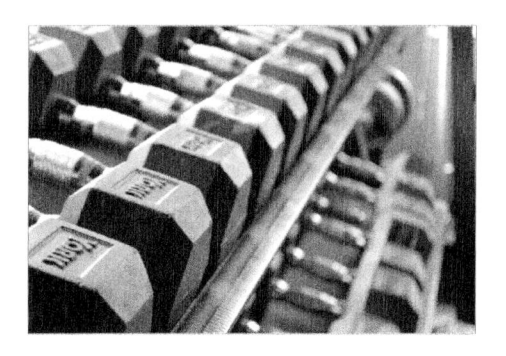

Strength Phase #2

So, you want to increase your strength as your annual goal.

In the second phase for strength you can change some exercise and push more weight. Maybe your legs or chest are not as strong as you would like: try to increase gradually the weight you lift, week after week.

> **Always keep track of your workouts**
>
> **You can subscribe to my webapp**
>
> **https://www.pt-manager.com**

Strength phase #2. Section 1. Week 1
Perceived effort level 8, add weight each set.

DAY	MUSCLES	EXERCISES
Monday	Full Body	Bench press [3 sets @ 5-6 RM] Military press [3 sets @ 15-6 RM] Low pulley row [3 sets @ 5-6 RM] Dumbbell curl [3 sets @ 5-6 RM] Cable pushdown [3 sets @ 5-6 RM] Leg curl [3 sets @ 5-6 RM] Squat [3 sets @ 5-6 RM] Crunch [3 sets @ 15-20RM]
Tuesday	Rest	
Wednesday	Full Body	Bench press [3 sets @ 5-6 RM] Military press [3 sets @ 15-6 RM] Low pulley row [3 sets @ 5-6 RM] Dumbbell curl [3 sets @ 5-6 RM] Cable pushdown [3 sets @ 5-6 RM] Leg curl [3 sets @ 5-6 RM] Squat [3 sets @ 5-6 RM] Crunch [3 sets @ 15-20RM]
Thursday	Rest	
Friday	Full Body	Bench press [3 sets @ 5-6 RM] Military press [3 sets @ 15-6 RM] Low pulley row [3 sets @ 5-6 RM] Dumbbell curl [3 sets @ 5-6 RM] Cable pushdown [3 sets @ 5-6 RM] Leg curl [3 sets @ 5-6 RM] Squat [3 sets @ 5-6 RM] Crunch [3 sets @ 15-20RM]
Saturday	Rest	Aerobic Activity
Sunday	Rest	

Strength phase #2. Section 1. Week 2
Perceived effort level 8, add weight each set.

DAY	MUSCLES	EXERCISES
Monday	Full Body	Bench press [3 sets @ 3-5 RM] Military press [3 sets @ 3-5 RM] Low pulley row [3 sets @ 3-5 RM] Dumbbell curl [3 sets @ 3-5 RM] Cable pushdown [3 sets @ 3-5 RM] Leg curl [3 sets @ 3-5 RM] Squat [3 sets @ 3-5 RM] Crunch [3 sets @ 15-20RM]
Tuesday	Rest	
Wednesday	Full Body	Bench press [3 sets @ 3-5 RM] Military press [3 sets @ 3-5 RM] Low pulley row [3 sets @ 3-5 RM] Dumbbell curl [3 sets @ 3-5 RM] Cable pushdown [3 sets @ 3-5 RM] Leg curl [3 sets @ 3-5 RM] Squat [3 sets @ 3-5 RM] Crunch [3 sets @ 15-20RM]
Thursday	Rest	
Friday	Full Body	Bench press [3 sets @ 3-5 RM] Military press [3 sets @ 3-5 RM] Low pulley row [3 sets @ 3-5 RM] Dumbbell curl [3 sets @ 3-5 RM] Cable pushdown [3 sets @ 3-5 RM] Leg curl [3 sets @ 3-5 RM] Squat [3 sets @ 3-5 RM] Crunch [3 sets @ 15-20RM]
Saturday	Rest	Aerobic Activity
Sunday	Rest	

Strength phase #2. Section 1. Week 3
Perceived effort level 8, add weight each set.

DAY	MUSCLES	EXERCISES
Monday	Full Body	Bench press [3 sets @ 1-3 RM] Military press [3 sets @ 1-3 RM] Low pulley row [3 sets @ 1-3 RM] Dumbbell curl [3 sets @ 1-3 RM] Cable pushdown [3 sets @ 1-3 RM] Leg curl [3 sets @ 1-3 RM] Squat [3 sets @ 1-3 RM] Crunch [3 sets @ 15-20RM]
Tuesday	Rest	
Wednesday	Full Body	Bench press [3 sets @ 1-3 RM] Military press [3 sets @ 1-3 RM] Low pulley row [3 sets @ 1-3 RM] Dumbbell curl [3 sets @ 1-3 RM] Cable pushdown [3 sets @ 1-3 RM] Leg curl [3 sets @ 1-3 RM] Squat [3 sets @ 1-3 RM] Crunch [3 sets @ 15-20RM]
Thursday	Rest	
Friday	Full Body	Bench press [3 sets @ 1-3 RM] Military press [3 sets @ 1-3 RM] Low pulley row [3 sets @ 1-3 RM] Dumbbell curl [3 sets @ 1-3 RM] Cable pushdown [3 sets @ 1-3 RM] Leg curl [3 sets @ 1-3 RM] Squat [3 sets @ 1-3 RM] Crunch [3 sets @ 15-20RM]
Saturday	Rest	Aerobic Activity
Sunday	Rest	

Strength phase #2. Section 1. Week 4
Perceived effort level 7.

DAY	MUSCLES	EXERCISES
Monday	Full Body	Bench press [3 sets @ 10-12 RM] Military press [3 sets @ 10-12 RM] Low pulley row [3 sets @ 10-12 RM] Dumbbell curl [3 sets @ 10-12 RM] Cable pushdown [3 sets @ 10-12 RM] Leg curl [3 sets @ 10-12 RM] Squat [3 sets @ 10-12 RM] Crunch [3 sets @ 15-20RM]
Tuesday	Rest	
Wednesday	Full Body	Bench press [3 sets @ 10-12 RM] Military press [3 sets @ 10-12 RM] Low pulley row [3 sets @ 10-12 RM] Dumbbell curl [3 sets @ 10-12 RM] Cable pushdown [3 sets @ 10-12 RM] Leg curl [3 sets @ 10-12 RM] Squat [3 sets @ 10-12 RM] Crunch [3 sets @ 15-20RM]
Thursday	Rest	
Friday	Full Body	Bench press [3 sets @ 10-12 RM] Military press [3 sets @ 10-12 RM] Low pulley row [3 sets @ 10-12 RM] Dumbbell curl [3 sets @ 10-12 RM] Cable pushdown [3 sets @ 10-12 RM] Leg curl [3 sets @ 10-12 RM] Squat [3 sets @ 10-12 RM] Crunch [3 sets @ 15-20RM]
Saturday	Rest	Aerobic Activity
Sunday	Rest	

Strength phase #2. Section 2. Week 5
Perceived effort level 8, add weight each set.

DAY	MUSCLES	EXERCISES
Monday	Upper Body	Bench press [3 sets @ 6-8 RM] Military press [3 sets @ 6-8 RM] Dumbbell flyes [3 sets @ 6-8 RM] Lat machine [3 sets @ 6-8 RM] Dumbbell curl [3 sets @ 6-8 RM] Cable pushdown [3 sets @ 6-8 RM]
Tuesday	Lower Body	Leg curl [3 sets @ 6-8 RM] Squat [3 sets @ 6-8 RM] Calf raise [3 sets @ 6-8 RM] Crunch [3 sets @ 15-20RM]
Wednesday	Rest	
Thursday	Upper Body	Bench press [3 sets @ 6-8 RM] Military press [3 sets @ 6-8 RM] Lateral raises [3 sets @ 6-8 RM] Lat machine [3 sets @ 6-8 RM] Dumbbell curl [3 sets @ 6-8 RM] Cable pushdown [3 sets @ 6-8 RM]
Friday	Lower Body	Leg curl [3 sets @ 6-8 RM] Squat [3 sets @ 6-8 RM] Calf raise [3 sets @ 6-8 RM] Crunch [3 sets @ 15-20RM]
Saturday	Rest	Aerobic Activity
Sunday	Rest	

Strength phase #2. Section 2. Week 6
Perceived effort level 8, add weight each set.

DAY	MUSCLES	EXERCISES
Monday	Upper Body	Bench press [3 sets @ 3-5 RM] Military press [3 sets @ 3-5 RM] Dumbbell flyes [3 sets @ 3-5 RM] Lat machine [3 sets @ 3-5 RM] Dumbbell curl [3 sets @ 3-5 RM] Cable pushdown [3 sets @ 3-5 RM]
Tuesday	Lower Body	Leg curl [3 sets @ 3-5 RM] Squat [3 sets @ 3-5 RM] Calf raise [3 sets @ 3-5 RM] Crunch [3 sets @ 15-20RM]
Wednesday	Rest	
Thursday	Upper Body	Bench press [3 sets @ 3-5 RM] Military press [3 sets @ 3-5 RM] Lateral raises [3 sets @3-5 RM] Lat machine [3 sets @ 3-5 RM] Dumbbell curl [3 sets @ 3-5 RM] Cable pushdown [3 sets @ 3-5 RM]
Friday	Lower Body	Leg curl [3 sets @ 3-5 RM] Squat [3 sets @ 3-5 RM] Calf raise [3 sets @ 3-5 RM] Crunch [3 sets @ 15-20RM]
Saturday	Rest	Aerobic Activity
Sunday	Rest	

Strength phase #2. Section 2. Week 7
Perceived effort level 9, add weight each set.

DAY	MUSCLES	EXERCISES
Monday	Upper Body	Bench press [3 sets @ 2-3 RM] Military press [3 sets @ 2-3 RM] Dumbbell flyes [3 sets @ 2-3 RM] Lat machine [3 sets @ 2-3 RM] Dumbbell curl [3 sets @ 2-3 RM] Cable pushdown [3 sets @ 2-3 RM]
Tuesday	Lower Body	Leg curl [3 sets @ 2-3 RM] Squat [3 sets @ 2-3 RM] Calf raise [3 sets @ 2-3 RM] Crunch [3 sets @ 15-20RM]
Wednesday	Rest	
Thursday	Upper Body	Bench press [3 sets @ 2-3 RM] Military press [3 sets @ 2-3 RM] Lateral raises [3 sets @ 2-3 RM] Lat machine [3 sets @ 2-3 RM] Dumbbell curl [3 sets @ 2-3 RM] Cable pushdown [3 sets @ 2-3 RM]
Friday	Lower Body	Leg curl [3 sets @ 2-3 RM] Squat [3 sets @ 2-3 RM] Calf raise [3 sets @ 2-3 RM] Crunch [3 sets @ 15-20RM]
Saturday	Rest	Aerobic Activity
Sunday	Rest	

Strength phase #2. Section 2. Week 8
Perceived effort level 7, add weight each set.

DAY	MUSCLES	EXERCISES
Monday	Upper Body	Bench press [3 sets @ 10-12 RM] Military press [3 sets @ 10-12 RM] Dumbbell flyes [3 sets @ 10-12RM] Lat machine [3 sets @ 10-12 RM] Dumbbell curl [3 sets @ 10-12 RM] Cable pushdown [3 sets @ 10-12 RM]
Tuesday	Lower Body	Leg curl [3 sets @ 10-12 RM] Squat [3 sets @ 10-12 RM] Calf raise [3 sets @ 10-12 RM] Crunch [3 sets @ 15-20RM]
Wednesday	Rest	
Thursday	Upper Body	Bench press [3 sets @ 10-12 RM] Military press [3 sets @ 10-12 RM] Dumbbell flyes [3 sets @ 10-12 RM] Lat machine [3 sets @ 10-12 RM] Dumbbell curl [3 sets @ 10-12 RM] Cable pushdown [3 sets @ 10-12 RM]
Friday	Lower Body	Leg curl [3 sets @ 10-12 RM] Squat [3 sets @ 10-12 RM] Calf raise [3 sets @ 10-12 RM] Crunch [3 sets @ 15-20RM]
Saturday	Rest	Aerobic Activity
Sunday	Rest	

Hypertrophy Phase #2

So, you want to increase your muscle mass as your yearly goal.

In this second phase for hypertrophy, you can change some exercise.

Maybe your legs are not as aspected: add more legs exercises.

Maybe your chest or back is not that of your dreams: do more exercises for that body part.

You should use a heavier weight than the first hypertrophy phase for each exercise.

> **Always keep track of your workout**
>
> **You can subscribe to my webapp**
>
> **https://www.pt-manager.com**

Hypertrophy phase #2. Mesocycle 1. Week 1.

DAY	MUSCLES	EXERCISES
Monday	Full Body	Dumbbell bench press [3 sets @ 10-12RM] Dumbbell military press [3 sets @ 10-12RM] Low pulley row [3 sets @ 10-12RM] Dumbbell curl [3 sets @ 10-12RM] Cable pushdown [3 sets @ 10-12RM] Leg curl [3 sets @ 10-12RM] Leg extension [3 sets @ 10-12RM] Crunch [3 sets @ 10-12RM] Calf raise [3 sets @ 10-12RM]
Tuesday	Rest	
Wednesday	Full Body	Dumbbell flyes [3 sets @ 10-12RM] Lateral raises [3 sets @ 10-12RM] Lat machine [3 sets @ 10-12RM] Dumbbell curl [3 sets @ 10-12RM] Cable pushdown [3 sets @ 10-12RM] Leg curl [3 sets @ 10-12RM] Leg extension [3 sets @ 10-12RM] Crunch [3 sets @ 10-12RM] Calf raise [3 sets @ 10-12RM]
Thursday	Rest	
Friday	Full Body	Dumbbell bench press [3 sets @ 10-12RM] Dumbbell military press [3 sets @ 10-12RM] Low pulley row [3 sets @ 10-12RM] Dumbbell curl [3 sets @ 10-12RM] Cable pushdown [3 sets @ 10-12RM] Leg curl [3 sets @ 10-12RM] Leg extension [3 sets @ 10-12RM] Crunch [3 sets @ 10-12RM] Calf raise [3 sets @ 10-12RM]
Saturday	Rest	Aerobic Activity
Sunday	Rest	

Hypertrophy phase #2. Mesocycle 1. Week 2.

DAY	MUSCLES	EXERCISES
Monday	Full Body	Dumbbell bench press [3 sets @ 8-10RM] Dumbbell military press [3 sets @ 1 8-10RM] Low pulley row [3 sets @ 8-10RM] Dumbbell curl [3 sets @ 8-10RM] Cable pushdown [3 sets @ 8-10RM] Leg curl [3 sets @ 8-10RM] Leg extension [3 sets @ 8-10RM] Crunch [3 sets @ 8-10RM] Calf raise [3 sets @ 8-10RM]
Tuesday	Rest	
Wednesday	Full Body	Dumbbell flyes [3 sets @ 8-10RM] Lateral raises [3 sets @ 8-10RM] Lat machine [3 sets @ 8-10RM] Dumbbell curl [3 sets @ 8-10RM] Cable pushdown [3 sets @ 8-10RM] Leg curl [3 sets @ 8-10RM] Leg extension [3 sets @ 8-10RM] Crunch [3 sets @ 8-10RM] Calf raise [3 sets @ 8-10RM]
Thursday	Rest	
Friday	Full Body	Dumbbell bench press [3 sets @ 8-10RM] Dumbbell military press [3 sets @ 1 8-10RM] Low pulley row [3 sets @ 8-10RM] Dumbbell curl [3 sets @ 8-10RM] Cable pushdown [3 sets @ 8-10RM] Leg curl [3 sets @ 8-10RM] Leg extension [3 sets @ 8-10RM] Crunch [3 sets @ 8-10RM] Calf raise [3 sets @ 8-10RM]
Saturday	Rest	
Sunday	Rest	

Hypertrophy phase #2. Mesocycle 1. Week 3.

Loads are increased and repetitions reduced, always with maximum control of movement. Recovery of 60 sec. between one set and another.

DAY	MUSCLES	EXERCISES
Monday	Full Body	Dumbbell bench press [3 sets @ 6-8RM] Dumbbell military press [3 sets @ 6-8RM] Low pulley row [3 sets @ 6-8RM] Dumbbell curl [3 sets @ 6-8 RM] Cable pushdown [3 sets @ 6-8RM] Leg curl [3 sets @ 6-8RM] Leg extension [3 sets @ 6-8RM] Crunch [3 sets @ 6-8RM] Calf raise [3 sets @ 6-8RM]
Tuesday	Rest	
Wednesday	Full Body	Dumbbell flyes [3 sets @ 6-8RM] Lateral raises [3 sets @ 6-8RM] Lat machine [3 sets @ 6-8RM] Dumbbell curl [3 sets @ 6-8RM] Cable pushdown [3 sets @ 6-8RM] Leg curl [3 sets @ 6-8RM] Leg extension [3 sets @ 6-8RM] Crunch [3 sets @ 6-8RM] Calf raise [3 sets @ 6-8RM]
Thursday	Rest	
Friday	Full Body	Dumbbell bench press [3 sets @ 6-8RM] Dumbbell military press [3 sets @ 6-8RM] Low pulley row [3 sets @ 6-8RM] Dumbbell curl [3 sets @ 6-8 RM] Cable pushdown [3 sets @ 6-8RM] Leg curl [3 sets @ 6-8RM] Leg extension [3 sets @ 6-8RM] Crunch [3 sets @ 6-8RM] Calf raise [3 sets @ 6-8RM]
Saturday	Rest	Aerobic Activity
Sunday	Rest	

Hypertrophy phase #2. Mesocycle 1. Week 4.
Lower the weights, increase repetitions, rest 45-60''

DAY	MUSCLES	EXERCISES
Monday	Full Body	Dumbbell bench press [3 sets @ 10-12RM] Dumbbell military press [3 sets @ 10-12RM] Low pulley row [3 sets @ 10-12RM] Dumbbell curl [3 sets @ 10-12RM] Cable pushdown [3 sets @ 10-12RM] Leg curl [3 sets @ 10-12RM] Leg extension [3 sets @ 10-12RM] Crunch [3 sets @ 10-12RM] Calf raise [3 sets @ 10-12RM]
Tuesday	Rest	
Wednesday	Full Body	Dumbbell flyes [3 sets @ 10-12RM] Lateral raises [3 sets @ 10-12RM] Lat machine [3 sets @ 10-12RM] Dumbbell curl [3 sets @ 10-12RM] Cable pushdown [3 sets @ 10-12RM] Leg curl [3 sets @ 10-12RM] Leg extension [3 sets @ 10-12RM] Crunch [3 sets @ 10-12RM] Calf raise [3 sets @ 10-12RM]
Thursday	Rest	
Friday	Full Body	Dumbbell bench press [3 sets @ 10-12RM] Dumbbell military press [3 sets @ 10-12RM] Low pulley row [3 sets @ 10-12RM] Dumbbell curl [3 sets @ 10-12RM] Cable pushdown [3 sets @ 10-12RM] Leg curl [3 sets @ 10-12RM] Leg extension [3 sets @ 10-12RM] Crunch [3 sets @ 10-12RM] Calf raise [3 sets @ 10-12RM]
Saturday	Rest	Aerobic Activity
Sunday	Rest	

Hypertrophy phase #2. Mesocycle 2. Week 5.

DAY	MUSCLES	EXERCISES
Monday	Chest, Back, Legs, Abs	Dumbbell bench press [4 sets @ 10-12RM] Dumbbell flyes [4 sets @ 10-12RM] Low pulley row [4 sets @ 10-12RM] Leg curl [4 sets @ 10-12RM] Crunch [4 sets @ 10-12RM]
Tuesday	Shoulders, Legs, Abs	Military press [4 sets @ 10-12RM] Lateral raises [4 sets @ 10-12RM] Rear lateral raises [4 sets @ 10-12RM] Leg extension [4 sets @ 10-12RM] Leg Press [4 sets @ 10-12RM] Calf raise [4 sets @ 10-12RM] Crunch [4 sets @ 10-12RM]
Wednesday	Arms, Abs	Dumbbell curl [3 sets @ 10-12RM] Cable pushdown [3 sets @ 10-12RM] Crunch [4 sets @ 10-12RM]
Thursday	Chest, Back, Legs, Abs	Dumbbell bench press [4 sets @ 10-12RM] Dumbbell flyes [4 sets @ 10-12RM] Lat machine [4 sets @ 10-12RM] Leg curl [4 sets @ 10-12RM] Crunch [4 sets @ 10-12RM]
Friday	Shoulders, Legs, Abs	Military press [4 sets @ 10-12RM] Lateral raises [4 sets @ 10-12RM] Rear lateral raises [4 sets @ 10-12RM] Leg extension [4 sets @ 10-12RM] Leg Press [4 sets @ 10-12RM] Calf raise [4 sets @ 10-12RM] Crunch [4 sets @ 10-12RM]
Saturday	Rest	Aerobic Activity
Sunday	Rest	

Hypertrophy phase #2. Mesocycle 2. Week 6.
Increase weights, rest 60-90''

DAY	MUSCLES	EXERCISES
Monday	Chest, Back, Legs, Abs	Dumbbell bench press [4 sets @ 8-10RM] Dumbbell flyes [4 sets @ 8-10RM] Low pulley row [4 sets @ 8-10RM] Leg curl [4 sets @ 8-10RM] Crunch [4 sets @ 15-20RM]
Tuesday	Shoulders, Legs, Abs	Military press [4 sets @ 8-10RM] Lateral raises [4 sets @ 8-10RM] Rear lateral raises [4 sets @ 8-10RM] Leg extension [4 sets @ 8-10RM] Leg Press [4 sets @ 8-10RM] Calf raise [4 sets @ 8-10RM] Crunch [4 sets @ 15-20RM]
Wednesday	Arms, Abs	Dumbbell curl [4 sets @ 8-10RM] Cable pushdown [4 sets @ 8-10RM] Crunch [4 sets @ 8-10RM]
Thursday	Chest, Back, Legs, Abs	Dumbbell bench press [4 sets @ 8-10RM] Dumbbell flyes [4 sets @ 8-10RM] Lat machine [4 sets @ 8-10RM] Leg curl [4 sets @ 8-10RM] Crunch [4 sets @ 15-20RM]
Friday	Shoulders, Legs, Abs	Military press [4 sets @ 8-10RM] Lateral raises [4 sets @ 8-10RM] Rear lateral raises [4 sets @ 8-10RM] Leg extension [4 sets @ 8-10RM] Leg Press [4 sets @ 8-10RM] Calf raise [4 sets @ 8-10RM] Crunch [4 sets @ 15-20RM]
Saturday	Rest	Aerobic Activity
Sunday	Rest	

Hypertrophy phase #2. Mesocycle 2. Week 7.
Increase sets using high weights, rest 60-90''

DAY	MUSCLES	EXERCISES
Monday	Chest, Back, Legs, Abs	Dumbbell bench press [5 sets @ 8-10 RM] Dumbbell flyes [5 sets @ 8-10 RM] Low pulley row [5 sets @ 8-10 RM] Leg curl [5 sets @ 8-10 RM] Crunch [4 sets @ 15-20 RM]
Tuesday	Shoulders, Legs, Abs	Military press [5 sets @ 8-10 RM] Lateral raises [5 sets @ 8-10 RM] Rear lateral raises [5 sets @ 8-10 RM] Leg extension [5 sets @ 8-10 RM] Leg Press [4 sets @ 8-10RM] Calf raise [5 sets @ 8-10 RM] Crunch [4 sets @ 15-20RM]
Wednesday	Arms, Abs	Dumbbell curl [5 sets @ 8-10RM] Cable pushdown [5 sets @ 8-10RM] Crunch [4 sets @ 15-20RM]
Thursday	Chest, Back, Legs, Abs	Dumbbell bench press [5 sets @ 8-10 RM] Dumbbell flyes [5 sets @ 8-10 RM] Lat machine [5 sets @ 8-10 RM] Leg curl [5 sets @ 8-10 RM] Crunch [4 sets @ 15-20 RM]
Friday	Shoulders, Legs, Abs	Military press [5 sets @ 8-10 RM] Lateral raises [5 sets @ 8-10 RM] Rear lateral raises [5 sets @ 8-10 RM] Leg extension [5 sets @ 8-10 RM] Leg Press [4 sets @ 8-10RM] Calf raise [5 sets @ 8-10 RM] Crunch [4 sets @ 15-20RM]
Saturday	Rest	Aerobic Activity
Sunday	Rest	

Hypertrophy phase #2. Mesocycle 2. Week 8.
Lower weights, increase repetitions, rest 45-60''

DAY	MUSCLES	EXERCISES
Monday	Chest, Back, Legs, Abs	Dumbbell bench press [4 sets @ 15-20RM] Dumbbell flyes [4 sets @ 15-20RM] Low pulley row [4 sets @ 15-20RM] Leg curl [4 sets @ 15-20RM] Crunch [4 sets @ 15-20RM]
Tuesday	Shoulders, Legs, Abs	Military press [4 sets @ 15-20RM] Lateral raises [4 sets @ 15-20RM] Rear lateral raises [4 sets @ 15-20RM] Leg extension [4 sets @ 15-20RM] Leg Press [4 sets @ 15-20RM] Calf raise [4 sets @ 15-20RM] Crunch [4 sets @ 15-20RM]
Wednesday	Arms, Abs	Dumbbell curl [3 sets @ 15-20RM] Cable pushdown [3 sets @ 15-20RM] Crunch [4 sets @ 15-20RM]
Thursday	Chest, Back, Legs, Abs	Dumbbell bench press [4 sets @ 15-20RM] Dumbbell flyes [4 sets @ 15-20RM] Lat machine [4 sets @ 15-20RM] Leg curl [4 sets @ 15-20RM] Crunch [4 sets @ 15-20RM]
Friday	Shoulders, Legs, Abs	Military press [4 sets @ 15-20RM] Lateral raises [4 sets @ 15-20RM] Rear lateral raises [4 sets @ 15-20RM] Leg extension [4 sets @ 15-20RM] Leg Press [4 sets @ 15-20RM] Calf raise [4 sets @ 15-20RM] Crunch [4 sets @ 15-20RM]
Saturday	Rest	Aerobic Activity
Sunday	Rest	

Hypertrophy phase #2. Mesocycle 3. Week 9.
Superset and triset. Rest di 60-90''

DAY	MUSCLES	EXERCISES
Monday	Chest, Back, Legs, Abs	Dumbbell bench press [4 sets @ 8-10 RM] superset with Dumbbell flyes [4 sets @ 8-10 RM] Low pulley row [4 sets @ 8-10 RM] Leg curl [4 sets @ 8-10 RM] Crunch [4 sets @ 15-20 RM]
Tuesday	Shoulders, Legs, Abs	Military press [4 sets @ 8-10 RM] triset with Lateral raises [4 sets @ 8-10 RM] e Rear lateral raises [4 sets @ 8-10 RM] Leg extension [4 sets @ 8-10 RM] superset with Leg Press [4 sets @ 8-10RM] Calf raise [4 sets @ 8-10 RM] Crunch [4 sets @ 15-20RM]
Wednesday	Arms, Abs	Dumbbell curl [4 sets @ 8-10RM] Cable pushdown [4 sets @ 8-10RM] Crunch [4 sets @ 15-20RM]
Thursday	Chest, Back, Legs, Abs	Dumbbell bench press [4 sets @ 8-10 RM] superset with Dumbbell flyes [4 sets @ 8-10 RM] Lat machine [4 sets @ 8-10 RM] Leg curl [4 sets @ 8-10 RM] Crunch [4 sets @ 15-20 RM]
Friday	Shoulders, Legs, Abs	Military press [4 sets @ 8-10 RM] triset with Lateral raises [4 sets @ 8-10 RM] e Rear lateral raises [4 sets @ 8-10 RM] Leg extension [4 sets @ 8-10 RM] superset with Leg Press [4 sets @ 8-10RM] Calf raise [4 sets @ 8-10 RM] Crunch [4 sets @ 15-20RM]
Saturday	Rest	Aerobic Activity
Sunday	Rest	

Hypertrophy phase #2. Mesocycle 3. Week 10.

DAY	MUSCLES	EXERCISES
Monday	Chest, Back, Legs, Abs	Dumbbell bench press [5 sets @ 8-10 RM] superset with Dumbbell flyes [5 sets @ 8-10 RM] Low pulley row [5 sets @ 8-10 RM] Leg curl [5 sets @ 8-10 RM] Crunch [4 sets @ 15-20 RM]
Tuesday	Shoulders, Legs, Abs	Military press [5 sets @ 8-10 RM] triset with Lateral raises [5 sets @ 8-10 RM] c Rear lateral raises [5 sets @ 8-10 RM] Leg extension [5 sets @ 8-10 RM] superset Leg Press [4 sets @ 8-10RM] Calf raise [5 sets @ 8-10 RM] Crunch [4 sets @ 15-20RM]
Wednesday	Arms, Abs	Dumbbell curl [5 sets @ 8-10RM] Cable pushdown [5 sets @ 8-10RM] Crunch [4 sets @ 15-20RM]
Thursday	Chest, Back, Legs, Abs	Dumbbell bench press [5 sets @ 8-10 RM] superset with Dumbbell flyes [5 sets @ 8-10 RM] Lat machine[5 sets @ 8-10 RM] Leg curl [5 sets @ 8-10 RM] Crunch [4 sets @ 15-20 RM]
Friday	Shoulders, Legs, Abs	Military press [5 sets @ 8-10 RM] triset with Lateral raises [5 sets @ 8-10 RM] c Rear lateral raises [5 sets @ 8-10 RM] Leg extension [5 sets @ 8-10 RM] superset with Leg Press [4 sets @ 8-10RM] Calf raise [5 sets @ 8-10 RM] Crunch [4 sets @ 15-20RM]
Saturday	Rest	Aerobic Activity
Sunday	Rest	

Hypertrophy phase #2. Mesocycle 3. Week 11.
Increase weight. Rest 90-120''

DAY	MUSCLES	EXERCISES
Monday	Chest, Back, Legs, Abs	Dumbbell bench press [4 sets @ 6-8 RM] superset with Dumbbell flyes [4 sets @ 6-8 RM] Low pulley row [4 sets @ 6-8 RM] Leg curl [4 sets @ 6-8 RM] Crunch [4 sets @ 15-20 RM]
Tuesday	Shoulders, Legs, Abs	Military press [4 sets @ 6-8 RM] triset with Lateral raises [4 sets @ 6-8 RM] e Rear lateral raises [4 sets @ 6-8 RM] Leg extension [4 sets @ 6-8 RM] superset with Leg Press [4 sets @ 6-8 RM] Calf raise [4 sets @ 6-8 RM] Crunch [4 sets @ 15-20RM]
Wednesday	Arms, Abs	Dumbbell curl [4 sets @ 6-8 RM] Cable pushdown [4 sets @ 6-8 RM] Crunch [4 sets @ 15-20RM]
Thursday	Chest, Back, Legs, Abs	Dumbbell bench press [4 sets @ 6-8 RM] superset with Dumbbell flyes [4 sets @ 6-8 RM] Lat machine [4 sets @ 6-8 RM] Leg curl [4 sets @ 6-8 RM] Crunch [4 sets @ 15-20 RM]
Friday	Shoulders, Legs, Abs	Military press [4 sets @ 6-8 RM] triset with Lateral raises [4 sets @ 6-8 RM] e Rear lateral raises [4 sets @ 6-8 RM] Leg extension [4 sets @ 6-8 RM] superset with Leg Press [4 sets @ 6-8 RM] Calf raise [4 sets @ 6-8 RM] Crunch [4 sets @ 15-20RM]
Saturday	Rest	Aerobic Activity
Sunday	Rest	

Hypertrophy phase #2. Mesocycle 3. Week 12.
Lower weight. Rest 60-90''

DAY	MUSCLES	EXERCISES
Monday	Chest, Back, Legs, Abs	Dumbbell bench press [4 sets @ 15-20RM] Dumbbell flyes [4 sets @ 15-20RM] Low pulley row [4 sets @ 15-20RM] Leg curl [4 sets @ 15-20RM] Crunch [4 sets @ 15-20RM]
Tuesday	Shoulders, Legs, Abs	Military press [4 sets @ 15-20RM] Lateral raises [4 sets @ 15-20RM] Rear lateral raises [4 sets @ 15-20RM] Leg extension [4 sets @ 15-20RM] Leg Press [4 sets @ 15-20RM] Calf raise [4 sets @ 15-20RM] Crunch [4 sets @ 15-20RM]
Wednesday	Arms, Abs	Dumbbell curl [3 sets @ 15-20RM] Cable pushdown [3 sets @ 15-20RM] Crunch [4 sets @ 15-20RM]
Thursday	Chest, Back, Legs, Abs	Dumbbell bench press [4 sets @ 15-20RM] Dumbbell flyes [4 sets @ 15-20RM] Lat machine [4 sets @ 15-20RM] Leg curl [4 sets @ 15-20RM] Crunch [4 sets @ 15-20RM]
Friday	Shoulders, Legs, Abs	Military press [4 sets @ 15-20RM] Lateral raises [4 sets @ 15-20RM] Rear lateral raises [4 sets @ 15-20RM] Leg extension [4 sets @ 15-20RM] Leg Press [4 sets @ 15-20RM] Calf raise [4 sets @ 15-20RM] Crunch [4 sets @ 15-20RM]
Saturday	Rest	Aerobic Activity
Sunday	Rest	

Aerobic Activity

As someone may have noticed, I have not included in my program specific times in which to perform an aerobic activity such as running or jumping rope or the treadmill. In order to build muscle mass, aerobic activity is useless. On the other hand, it can be useful in cases of weight loss or muscle definition that may follow a so-called "mass" phase, because it allows, in the case of activity prolonged for a certain time, to consume more calories than weight lifting. And obviously the more km you run, the greater the energy consumption. A moderate speed run is usually recommended, making sure you keep your heart rate between 65% to 80% of your maximum heart rate.

This maximum heart rate can be obtained in a rough but indicative way with the following formula:
FCMax = 220 - age.

The minimum time of aerobic activity usually recommended is at least 20 minutes per session. This may have a benefit in terms of physical condition and metabolic improvement.

In any case, you do not lose weight while doing physical activity but through a calorie deficit over time. Aerobic activity helps this process because it increases the consumption of calories and therefore allows the aforementioned caloric deficit to be increased.

To get an idea of the role of aerobic activity in weight loss, we can use some useful formulas developed over time by sports science researcher: Energy expenditure (KCal) = 1kcal x kg of weight x km traveled (Arcelli formula). For example 1kcal x 75kg (weight) x 10 Km =

750kcal consumed. Science has established the percentages of carbohydrate and fat used as a function of the percentage of maximum heart rate, through the respiratory quotient and the Vomax. A heart rate below 80% of the maximum heart rate leads us to burn an average of 70% of carbohydrates and 30% of fat. Going back to our example, to know the amount of kcal of fat burned we need to calculate 30% of 750 kcal, which is 225 kcal. One gram of fat corresponds to 9 kcal but in the human body the fat mass (adipocyte) is combined with water for which 1kg of body fat represents about 7,000 kcal and not 9,000 kcal. So in practice 1 gram of body fat corresponds to 7kcal. In practice, in the training session of our example 225kcal / 7 = 32.2 gr were consumed. of fat. For example, to lose 3 kilos and 220 grams (32.2 grams * 1000 grams (1Kg)), while keeping all other parameters unchanged, you have to run for 10,000 km. It is clear that to obtain results in terms of weight loss, one cannot ignore a diet that generates a caloric deficit, compared to the energy consumption that one is used to, that is protracted over time. And this is true regardless of the type of diet in vogue in a given historical period. You can also lose weight by eating more carbohydrates if your overall calorie intake is lower than your energy consumption.

How to continue

It all depends on your goals. In general, for those looking for greater strength it is good to enter at least two periods of strength during the year, as we have seen before. After the period dedicated to strength it is good to insert a period of recovery or hypertrophy, that is, it is good to allow the body to recover from the stress of the period with high loads.

If, on the other hand, hypertrophy is your goal, you can continue alternating 12 weeks of hypertrophy like those described above with 4 weeks of recovery, decreasing the load and increasing the metabolic work. In every stage dedicated to hypertrophy you can favoring the deficient muscle groups, working them more.

Visit www.fitnessedintorni.it for bonus materials
or
write
info@fitnessedintorni.it
for advice on training and healthy eating

Lockdown

This book assumes that the gyms are open and therefore exercises with some typical gym machines are proposed.

In periods of lockdown, we can replace most of the exercises with some equipment that we can keep or already have at home: a basic set includes a flat bench that is also reclining, one or more sets of dumbbells, a pull-up bar. All items are easily purchased new or used. The most important thing is to have enough weights to stimulate muscle growth. It is true that the lack of adequate weight can be replaced with an increase in the number of repetitions, but only to a certain point. A scarce movement is better than no movement, but to increase strength you need to lift weights that are able to push the muscle to adjust its capacity to the weight lifted.

More complex is the work to be done outside the gym relating to the legs. Usually, this muscle group requires more weight. We have to replace the machines such as leg press, leg extension and leg curl with squats and lunges, increasing the number of repetitions and using the dumbbells.

If we really can't get any equipment we can perform free body exercises such as push-ups, crunches, squats, lunges, which at least allow us to keep fit. In this case, I recommend that you create a plan that involves performing 100 push-ups per day, 100 bodyweight squats and 100 crunches: with half an hour a day you will feel like lions! If you are not trained enough, set yourself the goal of reaching that level after one or two months, starting from where you are and increasing by 10 repetitions every day.

For specific advice related to your situation you can write to me to book an interview **info@fitnessedintorni.it**. On www.fitnessedintorni.it you will find welcome offers.

See you soon and Up the Irons *

* For Heavy Metal Freaks

For a complete course on bodybuilding and body recomposition check out my book on Amazon
https://www.amazon.com/dp/B08RK235ZX

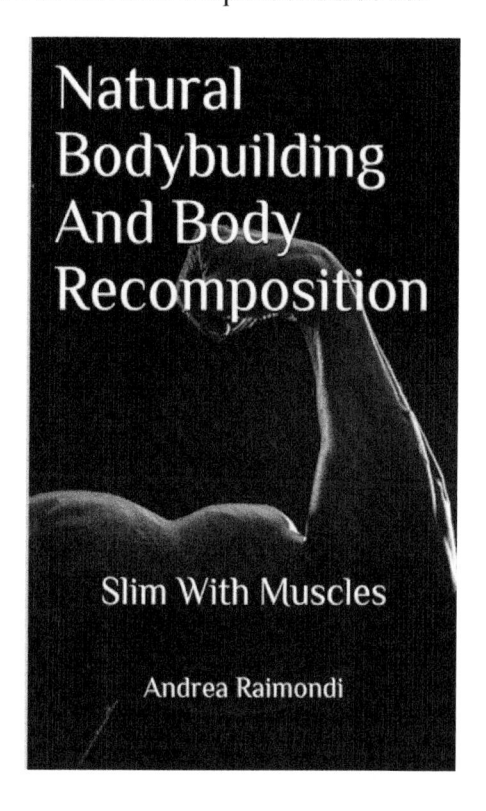

Motivation

Taken from my "Natural Bodybuilding and Body Recomposition"

Build a stronger, more muscular and healthier body takes time, it takes dedication, it takes patience. You have to find the strength within **yourself** to train even when everything tells you to let it go. After all, we all have dozens of distractions. Many things tell us to choose the most comfortable way and the body itself tends to inaction. To choose the most comfortable way.

We need motivation and a positive mental approach. In fact, as in all other aspects of life, the role of the mind is fundamental to achieving any result. You must have the will not to give up your training routine. And the will must also be trained through a positive mental focus. But what does it mean? It means going beyond the difficulties of the moment and looking at the final goal, at building muscle mass, at the physique you want to have, and always believing that it is achievable. For this, it is necessary to set goals and plan the path to achieve them.

Set goals

Having a goal is like seeing a lighthouse during an offshore storm. It allows you to stay on course towards what you want to be or become. This is why it is important to establish what you want to achieve: more muscles? less fat? It is also important to give yourself a reasonable time to get it: I can't think of putting on 20 kg of muscle in a year of training, I can't think of losing 20 kg in a month without problems. And it is better to set the goal precisely: I want to lose 10 kg in six months, I want to have 5 kg more muscle in a year. In this way, it will be easier to measure whether the direction taken is the correct one, the one that leads to the achievement of the goal. It will be easier to measure progress or stalls and take action accordingly. Once the goal has been established, this must always be remembered at every training session, whenever you don't want to train, and even when you don't seem to get the desired results. You must never stray from your goal. In defining the goal, it is necessary to go into details, break down the goal into many smaller, more easily achievable phases, create monthly, weekly, daily routines. This way you can set measurable goals for each period, for example losing 0.5 kg per week means 12 kg in 6 months, and focus on achieving this weekly goal. You must always remember that in body recomposition the time factor counts, you must give your body time to adapt to the new situation and give it time to break homeostasis. You must want to achieve the goal, so ask yourself what you **REALLY** want to achieve. And everything will become easier. Then take action, prepare a training plan, and follow it consistently. The confidence gained in seeing constant small improvements will give you the strength and energy to continue towards the goal.

Maximum concentration

When training, you should focus on the movement you are doing, feel which muscle is contracting, check if the posture is correct, in short, you must try to be focused on yourself.

Continuous experimentation

You have created your own plan or used one of those provided in the book and you follow it faithfully, with constancy and discipline, but may it happen that in a training session you feel more tired or bored from the usual routine? It is time to try something new, try an exercise that you haven't done for a long time or that you have never done, change the load, increase or decrease the repetitions.

This way can help you resume your usual pattern in the following days with greater vigor.

Because it is important to complete the training schedule for the set period without constantly changing exercises: you need to build willpower to stay fixed on the established course.

Push hard

We can combine it with concentration: the more concentrated you are, the more you can push hard: completing a work session that is training does not mean you must break the muscle fibers every time; it means giving your best for how you feel that day: if you feel tired because you slept little or ate badly, give your best in those conditions, but never give up, never give up on the planned training.

For a complete course on bodybuilding and body recomposition check out my book on Amazon
https://www.amazon.com/dp/B08RK235ZX

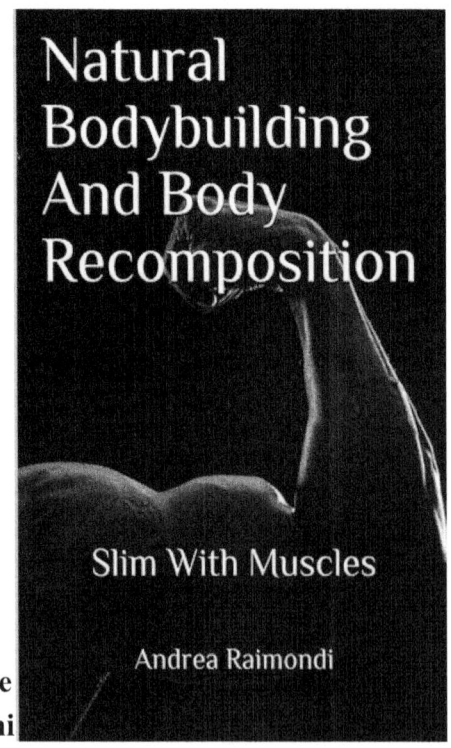

info@fitnessedintorni.it

www.fitnessedintorni.it

www.pt-manager.com

BONUS Lunch-time Workout

Many of us have to manage many responsibilities between family and work and time for training is left among the last things to do.

In these cards, I propose a workout to be carried out during the lunch break every working day. It is a short workout, about 35-40 minutes but following the principles of the progression of loads and keeping recoveries under one minute can give great results.

In this example we will train the chest and shoulders 2 times a week, the legs 5 times, and the back 4 times.

Modify the type of exercises according to your needs: you can decide, for example, to train the chest or shoulders more and train less back and legs.

Card to be carried out for 12 weeks, after the first 4 weeks increase the loads bringing the reps to 10 per set after another 4 weeks return to lower the load and increasing the repetitions. Repeat the cycle throughout the year.

Example Week Plan

DAY	MUSCLES	EXERCISES
Monday	Chest, Back, Legs, Abs	Dumbbell bench press [4 sets @ 12RM] Low pulley row [4 sets @ 12RM] Leg extension [4 sets @ 12RM] Crunch [2 sets @ 30 reps]
Tuesday	Shoulders, Legs, Back, Abs	Military press [4 sets @ 12RM] Lateral raises [4 sets @ 12RM] Lat Machine [4 sets @ 12RM] Leg curl [4 sets @ 12RM] Crunch [4 sets @ 30 reps]
Wednesday	Arms, Legs, Abs	Dumbbell curl [4 sets @ 12RM] Cable pushdown [4 sets @ 12RM] Leg Press [4 sets @ 20 RM] Crunch [4 sets @ 15-20RM]
Thursday	Chest, Back, Legs, Abs	Dumbbell bench press [4 sets @ 12RM] Low pulley row [4 sets @ 12RM] Leg extension [4 sets @ 12RM] Crunch [2 sets @ 30 reps]
Friday	Shoulders, Legs, Back, Abs	Military press [4 sets @ 12RM] Lateral raises [4 sets @ 12RM] Lat Machine [4 sets @ 12RM] Leg curl [4 sets @ 12RM] Crunch [4 sets @ 30 reps]
Saturday	Rest	Aerobic Activity
Sunday	Rest	

Visit www.fitnessedintorni.it for bonus materials
or
write
info@fitnessedintorni.it
for advice on training and healthy eating